FIBROMYALGIA:
UNRAVELLING THE MYSTERIES OF THE DIS-EASE

FIBROMYALGIA:
UNRAVELLING THE MYSTERIES
OF THE DIS-EASE

BARBARA A. KEDDY R.N. (ret), Ph.D.

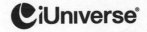 iUniverse®

FIBROMYALGIA: UNRAVELLING THE MYSTERIES OF THE DIS-EASE

iUniverse books may be ordered through booksellers or by contacting:

iUniverse
1663 Liberty Drive
Bloomington, IN 47403
www.iuniverse.com
844-349-9409

Because of the dynamic nature of the Internet, any web addresses or links contained in this book may have changed since publication and may no longer be valid. The views expressed in this work are solely those of the author and do not necessarily reflect the views of the publisher, and the publisher hereby disclaims any responsibility for them.

Any people depicted in stock imagery provided by Getty Images are models, and such images are being used for illustrative purposes only.
Certain stock imagery © Getty Images.

Library of Congress Control Number: 2022913265
ISBN: 978-1-6632-4239-6 (sc)
ISBN: 978-1-6632-4240-2 (e)

Print information available on the last page.

iUniverse rev. date: 07/12/2022

To Milt

Contents

Introduction

How this book came to be

Fibromyalgia syndrome (FMS) is a mysterious condition that affects millions. Because it is poorly understood by the medical establishment, it is difficult to find effective treatments. A great deal of fear surrounds fibromyalgia, as I know, sadly, from personal experience. I hope to confront some of these common fears and share as much information as I have in an effort to bring this chronic dis-ease into the light.

In the following pages, I explore theories I have developed based on my own experience of FMS that may be controversial to some but bring hope to others. They are not scientifically proven theories, but since no such things currently exist, I offer my own, those of others who live with FMS, and my extensive research into FMS and its treatment.

Fibromyalgia and its sidekick, chronic fatigue syndrome have been my constant companion for most of my life, though I didn't always know them by their names. Keeping these conditions hidden was how I survived my earlier life as I was ashamed of admitting I was often in a state of pain and fatigue. But to those close to me (mainly my spouse) I "complained" so often that guilt accompanied my many struggles. It wasn't until I began researching the topic of fibromyalgia in great detail over twenty years ago that I had a name for this invisible dis-ease. I wanted to learn more about my condition and to share what I was learning. After interviewing many other women with FMS —both formally with signed consent, and informally as occasions arose— I published my first book, *Women and Fibromyalgia: Living with an Invisible Dis-ease* in 2007 (iUniverse). I also began work on a now-defunct website where I posted blogs about my experiences with FMS; the comments I received from readers provided me with the inspiration to write this new book.

In hindsight, I regret that I wrote my first book in such an exclusionary style specifically focussing on women; I have learned that there are just as many men who suffer from this syndrome even though it is often labelled differently for them. This book is inclusive of all genders.

The many women and men who over many years have commented on my blogs have given me the courage to go out on a limb once more about what I believe to be the cause of this invisible condition. After a thorough review of both formal interviews and blogs I decided that a new book needed to be written as an update to the first. I also noted that books on FMS that were published after my 2007 book have not revealed much new information for me that coincides with my view about this invisible syndrome called fibromyalgia. Hence the need for another book.

To the readers of the blogs whose comments have added to my understanding of the daily hardships we suffer, often in silence, I give a heartfelt thank you. To those women I formally interviewed years ago, I hope that your syndrome has not worsened and I acknowledge your contribution to my evolved insights. To all of you who wrote replies to my blogs, your comments cannot be included here as I did not request permission from you to include them in a book. However, I thank you for trusting me with your stories. You are the experts on your own bodies and I have learned so much from you.

I am grateful to the experts and authors on pain I admired so long ago: Diane Jacobs, Bronnie Thompson, David Butler, and Lorimer Moseley, among a host of others who came along a little later in my epiphany. *Waking the Tiger: Healing Trauma* by Peter Levine (1997) is the book which began my quest to explore "the mystery of trauma." I am so thankful to all those neuroscientists uncovering the wonderous mechanisms of the brain. They have shown me the route to unravelling this mystery.

Perhaps I am wrong in my subjective analysis. I don't propose that I am *the* expert on this disorder as it is a very diffuse syndrome. I am instead writing what I believe is a reasonable, yet tentative explanation based upon personal experience and the experiences of many hundreds of others who have written to me over the years, those who suffer from fibromyalgia and chronic fatigue.

I am not a Buddhist, but Buddhist philosophy has been another guide for me throughout these past decades. Mindfulness and meditation have allowed me the opportunity to become self-reflective, which is key to an understanding of the difficult workings of the mind/ brain and the functioning of the central nervous system. To be living in the sequestered era of Covid-19 has also allowed me time for reflection that would otherwise not have been as fruitful.

As mentioned earlier, since I wrote my first book, times have changed and so has the discourse around gender identities. Now as never before, I finally refute the idea of women being the main gender of those who suffer from fibromyalgia. I acknowledge that the issues related to gender identities and gender fluidity are complex. Is a gay man not as vulnerable to this syndrome as a self-identified woman? Is a transitioned woman as likely to have this dis-ease? What about bisexual people or others who are non-binary? Those who identify as women are not only those who are heterosexual-identified females. I apologize for the years when *he* and *she* were the main gender pronouns we used in our discourse. All people are vulnerable to trauma, anxiety and depression, whether or not we are marginalized, racialized, or on the gender spectrum, resulting in a dis-ease which cannot be seen, but is still experienced.

Though the world has changed dramatically since I began publishing blog posts on FMS, I stand by the references in them that were new to me then and are still not outdated. These writings are like my memoir.

Many years ago, as a university professor teaching research methodology, I would often ask students some of the following questions: What is knowledge? Who creates it and for what purposes? To whom is it made available? What is the difference between (supposedly) objective science and personal, subjective, anecdotal experience? As mentioned earlier, this book does not pretend that what I put forward is scientific in the usual objective sense of the word. It is primarily about my own intuition, journey, and those of others who have had similar experiences like mine living with an invisible syndrome which cannot yet be scientifically explained. It is about our own lived experiences and the commonality of knowledge about how this dis-ease "feels" to us. I hope readers will find some of my ideas helpful, though I am not a physician and do not give medical advice that is outside my realm of expertise as a retired nurse. Specifically, the only advice I give is based upon public knowledge.

Some invisible conditions, for want of better labels are called fibromyalgia, chronic fatigue syndrome, post traumatic stress disorder, multiple chemical sensitivities, migraines and perhaps even "long Covid-19," although I know the inclusion of the last condition is unfounded and potentially controversial. I hope it becomes clearer as the stories emerge that I believe they are all closely related (excluding long Covid), and perhaps are all the same thing manifested in different ways, with similar symptoms.

When I first began writing about fibromyalgia it seemed life was somewhat "normal," whatever that meant before Covid. Some days were good, others not so good: ups and downs are common with fibromyalgia. Never could we have anticipated a worldwide pandemic when societies would be in a state of chronic anxiety and panic and routines were greatly disrupted. For those of us living in a state of near constant uncertainty and distress about our fibromyalgia disorder, Covid-19 has increased our ruminations about our health, as many of our FMS symptoms almost completely mimic those of Covid-19.

Until I was double-vaccinated, this fear accelerated every day. Later a booster vaccine was administered, followed by the arrival of a new variant; it never seemed to end. Living with a new norm of masking and distancing, I have now accepted that life will likely be more uncertain than ever before. This acceptance has brought a little measure of peace.

How I began my learning journey and where it has led me

In 1998, while on sabbatical at the University of British Columbia, I travelled to Galiano Island, B.C., for an appointment with a retired physician who specialized in fibromyalgia. I received the diagnosis which I had suspected for several years. For some reason I believed that a definite diagnosis from this reputable neurologist would legitimize my life-long dis-ease. It was official; I had fibromyalgia, he told me. This physician, who had practiced in Vancouver for many years, had set up an amazing space for a meditation retreat, while also continuing to consult with a few patients. His wife had fibromyalgia and together they ran the Centre, a calming, safe place that created a healing atmosphere. Here I met others with the same condition and began to slowly understand that those of us with fibromyalgia were very similar in personal characteristics.

After I returned to my office at UBC, I began the process of formally interviewing women who were fellow sufferers, interviews which formed the genesis of my first book. During this process, I learned that millions of us suffer from formally diagnosed or undiagnosed fibromyalgia and wonder where to find helpful information.

I have not read a book, article or blog specifically about fibromyalgia that has given me all the answers I needed. It is not my intent to detail those writings which often cite symptoms, the trigger points that help in a diagnosis, or to present alternative therapies that are often somewhat outlandish. Details about medications that are prescribed, or older references that are often not helpful would interfere with the journalistic style of this book.

Rather, this is a book based upon a review of the 130+ blog posts I wrote over a decade and the comments from readers for whom I have the utmost respect and learned so much from. The people who took the time to comment on my blogs and share their stories of pain, frustration and confusion as well as their courage are integral to my views in this book. Those of us with this mysterious condition have been silenced too long.

Reviewing all of this information has been a fascinating experience in and of itself. I find myself travelling back in time, observing the thoughts and questions I once had and still do have, while wondering about those who sent me such tales of sadness, hope, and heroism while managing to live their lives to the best of their ability.

To those who do not believe that this syndrome even exists, I invite you to spend a week with someone who struggles with the challenges of everyday life while living with fibromyalgia. Its invisibility and the difficulty with diagnosis consistently lead to frustration and despair.

Are we forever doomed to suffer in silence? Going from physician to physician hoping for answers, subjecting ourselves to multiple tests, and trying one medication after another do not usually provide satisfactory answers or solutions. The old trigger point test of pressing on certain points of the body is not helpful as we are usually sore all over and pain radiates from one area to another in a non- systematic way. There isn't any medical test which can determine with certainty that one has fibromyalgia.

I have learned so much over the past two decades from many sources: experts on the brain, the "culprit" in this mystery, have taught me about its ability to change, and therapists have shared valuable insights that have resulted in different pathways to explore. Unbelievably wonderful but difficult books about the neuroplasticity of the brain, have led me to understand the relationship of multiple chemical sensitivities (MCS), post traumatic stress disorder (PTSD), fibromyalgia (FMS) and chronic fatigue (CFS) how they all seem to be related to one another. Each have given me interesting insights that allowed me to develop a potential theory about their cause. I have learned about the type of person who develops fibromyalgia, but I realize that many other health professionals and scientists can challenge my theory. I recognize that I write from a position of white, heterosexual, first world privilege and I acknowledge I do not represent all who suffer from fibromyalgia whose life circumstances differ dramatically from mine. Unlike FMS sufferers in other parts of the world, I have the luxury of a bed at night and good food; I can speak about my pain and not be searching for a place to live or seeking my next meal.

In the few years before I retired, I was involved in research projects about the health of Black Nova Scotian women.[1] The women had many differences: race, age, economics and living in rural versus urban areas. With the several women I interviewed for the first book what we had in common was that we all suffered from fibromyalgia. The project culminated in that earlier book previously mentioned on fibromyalgia-*Women and Fibromyalgia Living with an Invisible Dis-ease.*

The experience of writing that book exemplified the various forms of discrimination faced by many in society. I myself have experienced sexism and ageism. I have also at one time been economically disadvantaged, but never homeless. All women have had covert or overt experiences of sexism. Unless we are lesbian/ gay / bi/trans/queer/genderfluid, we will not experience homophobia. I cannot then write about all of us with fibromyalgia as if we were universal human beings with similar life stories.

---

[1] Note that there is disagreement in Canada about which term, "African Canadian" or "Black", is preferable.

As mentioned elsewhere, I no longer focus on one gender; rather, I acknowledge gender fluidity and gender as a social construct. Hence while my view on fibromyalgia has not changed, it is no longer binary.

I think it is important to point out that FMS sufferers may live under circumstances that are unique to each of us in terms of race, gender, social class, education, geography, age, sexual/gender identity, physical and mental abilities, but we do have this one unifying struggle. We know what it is like to wake up each day to pain and crushing fatigue, as well as all the other challenges that go with this syndrome. Therefore, I ask of you to be tolerant of me if I write as though I can know about your daily challenges. I can only know that we do have one thing in common, that demon, fibromyalgia that lives with us and won't completely let go!

During the writing of my first book, I was guided to Elaine Aron's *The Highly Sensitive Person* (1996) and I have not looked back. I was no longer interested in a speculative cause for FMS that could be viral, bacterial, or hormonal, nor one that could be called a disease, but rather a syndrome which was the result of a personality type with specific life experiences. I was no longer just interested in the systems that eventually broke down in the person living with FMS, as they were not the cause but the result. Instead, I have concentrated on finding the root cause of FMS and the symptoms that ensue, and finally the ways in which this disorder can be managed for a better quality of life. I persist in believing my theory about the cause of FMS is the only one that makes sense of what has always seemed to be a mysterious and actual disease, rather than what it really is: a "dis-ease." I have never yet found anyone with fibromyalgia to dispute what I suggest are the causes of this syndrome. Those hundreds of readers who submitted comments and the women who spoke to me directly in formal interviews are in agreement with my theoretical approach to fibromyalgia. I have relied on their lived experiences, and my own.

The number of symptoms of FMS is vast and I cannot cover them all, but I will discuss those which are the most common. Symptoms are what most people want to discuss in support groups, on websites and in conversations. While dwelling too much on symptoms can be counterproductive, it is what unites us. In fact, these symptoms are often experienced by people who do not have fibromyalgia and I cannot prove that they are always due to this syndrome, but may perhaps be attributable to the minor irritations of everyday living. It is often difficult to separate rather inconsequential issues from serious manifestations of a disease.

Finally, the management of this condition rests with certain basic strategies that everyone can undertake to better their quality of life. They offer a degree of hope but rely on the individual to attempt a degree of control of our own lives, given our dis-abilities.

What I do not do is cite references in great detail unless they had appeared in a blog, nor present them in the usual academic fashion as I believe it is too distracting for the reader who often has little energy to spare. The references I do cite were included at the time of the writing over the past decade and are still relevant. I have also included newer ones for those who want to further their own research.

The unproven theory that I present over and over about causes may begin to become repetitive so I warn the reader in advance. I always call this syndrome a dis-ease, not a disease. Those whom I interviewed or sent comments to me all agreed, but some lapsed into the medical jargon of "disease".

Finally, a note on the structure of this book. It is written as a series of short blog-style essays, each on a topic relating to some aspect of living with fibromyalgia. These can be read in sequence or separately, as the reader prefers.

PART 1

CAUSES AND SYMPTOMS OF FIBROMYALGIA

The FMS personality

"If we can stay grounded and not get caught up in our
catastrophizing thoughts, we can begin to meet the
anxiety, and our circumstances, with equanimity"
– Andrew Safer

All people have psychic wounds and challenges we cannot see.
This is why fibromyalgia is *invisible*, and eventually becomes a chronic
malfunctioning of the central nervous system.

My theory of causation is that fibromyalgia will occur in specific
personality types:

1. The individual will be a highly-sensitive person, feeling things
    perhaps too deeply
2. The individual will be a highly anxious and/or a depressive person
    whose mind is rarely quiet
3. The individual will have suffered a difficult past with trauma that
    results in overt or hidden anxiety
4. The individual will be a hyper-vigilant person, that is, often
    experience a profound feeling of impending danger
5. The individual will have an easily aroused central nervous system
    (CNS), that is, the CNS is malfunctioning after prolonged anxiety
6. The individual will have triggers that bring on feelings of
    fearfulness, possibly panic attacks and chronic anxiety
7. The individual will be an overly empathetic person, often a
    caregiver and very intuitive
8. The individual will catastrophize easily

9. The individual will have been a high achiever, in a hurry, often impatient for things to be well organized
10. This individual will have full blown chronic fibromyalgia after a crisis such as an illness or accident, witnessing war, sexual or physical abuse, death, divorce or after exposure to real or potential violence. A pre-existing condition such as lupus or multiple sclerosis may also be present. (Note that currently just living through the Covid-19 pandemic, either having had it or losing someone who was a victim to the dreaded virus may result in fibromyalgia.)

Psychosomatic Disorder or Stored Memories?

"Trust one who has gone through it."
– Virgil

Writing that word "psychosomatic," in fact, even thinking about the word, makes me uncomfortable! Who wants to be labeled as one whose pain is thought to be "**JUST** in your head," implying it is not real? One of the women I interviewed in the first book, Monica (name changed) had the same feeling: "If you can actually have someone diagnose something, at least it's easier, rather than thinking it's all in your head because that's what I have been thinking for years and there are some doctors that have thought the same thing."

But before we go off into a tailspin about that demeaning-sounding phrase, I should begin by saying what I now believe "psychosomatic" to mean. It certainly does not suggest that those of us with fibromyalgia are hysterics who malinger just to get attention. But maybe our physical disorders are caused by traumatic emotions that are unconscious and deep-seated and **are** in our head (brain), reflected by the extreme tightening of our muscles causing the pain. Such emotions as intense fear, sadness, anxiety, and rage can be kept in a closed segment of our minds without taking them out to examine and work with consciously. After all, pain perceptions come from our body's nociceptors, (that is, pain receptors that respond to real or potentially damaging stimuli) funneled up to the brain. "Psychosomatic" does not mean that the pain and other symptoms are not real, but that they come from the brain in our stored memories.

3

The other term often used by health professionals is "psychogenesis," that is, the development of a physical disorder or illness resulting from psychic rather than physiological factors. Both terms are used to describe fibromyalgia.

Being female, economically disadvantaged, un-housed, of marginalized races or ethnic groups, disabled, or of a gender identity that differs from the majority, or anyone who has been victimized or abused in some way or has been taught to care for others to the exclusion of themselves...all of these factors can result in a plethora of thoughts and feelings that eventually evoke painful body experiences. We develop a hurricane of emotions. To add to our internal struggles, anxiety about war and climate change are current factors that most of us are fearful about. The state of the world can bring about flare-ups of this demon along with stored memories of earlier fears.

Some people with FMS can trace its beginnings to a definite event, like a surgery or a long illness. One of the women I interviewed for the first book, Bonnie, said, "I think it happened for me after my hysterectomy. But I think I had the signs of it before that time." Another woman, Mary, said of her FMS, "I date the onset to probably the time when my immune system took a dramatic hit from mono, but in general I attribute it to a lifetime of surviving high stress without respite".

Memories of pain, like that caused from surgery, accidents or abuse can become stored in our brains, inciting fear upon recall or finding ourselves in a situation that may unconsciously remind us of the one in which we were initially hurt. Because we learn by finding patterns in our experiences, our brain is very good at recognizing real or potential threats and sends us warnings to protect us from experiencing pain again. Thoughts of emotional or physical trauma become lodged in our brain (in the *amygdala* wherein lies the "flight or fight" response) and are expressed as disorders like pain in various parts of our bodies– that is what I mean by "psychosomatic." We store unpleasant memories in the unconscious part of the brain and when stress or excitement occurs, our nervous system is activated to either fight or take flight because of perceived danger.

As Dr. Peter Levine suggests in his book *Waking the Tiger: Healing Trauma*, there is a third automatic nervous system response: freezing, where the brain attempts to stop painful emotions at their source. The highly sensitive and overly empathetic person described in an earlier section may be particularly prone to this protective response, which leads us to wonder if years of freezing difficult emotions make this person more likely to develop fibromyalgia.

Studies on people with higher-than-average levels of empathy have shown thicker gray matter in the right frontal lobe of the brain where non-verbal abilities are located. Did the thickness evolve from our early years of socialization (learned empathy) or was the person born that way? If so, why is empathy so often associated with women? The authors of the empathy study suggest that higher levels of testosterone in men makes them less empathetic. Once again, in my search for answers on causes of FMS, I am left in a quandary. Is it caused by nature, nurture or both? How much is related to our environment and how much is biology? What else can contribute? Do trans women also become overly empathetic? I have more questions than answers.

Further, is there another reason for our psychic and physical pain? What if the pain from the unconscious part of the brain expresses itself with tension in a particular body part and that area becomes oxygen-deprived, causing pain? This is the view of Dr. John E. Sarno in his 2006 book *The Divided Mind: The Epidemic of Mind-Body Disorders* in which he discusses fibromyalgia in somewhat lengthy excerpts. If he is correct (and I am not sure about this), then do we have reason to believe that we have been disregarded or ignored by the health care system?

How do we reach our unconscious thoughts and rid ourselves of pain if they are truly frozen? Are these emotions actually the root cause of our condition? Does the body become oxygen deprived? Is fibromyalgia actually a physical disease as I have disputed? I always have more questions than answers.

Fibromyalgia, Sensitivity, and Anxiety

"My anxiety remains an unhealed wound that, at times, holds
me back and fills me with shame, but it may also be, at the same
time, a source of strength and a bestower of certain blessings."
– Scott Stossel

I believe fibromyalgia can be viewed as an extreme case of prolonged anxiety that begins in early life, perhaps in utero, and may even be genetically-inherited. Having read Daniel Smith's *Monkey Mind* and Scott Stossel's, *My Age of Anxiety* memoirs, along with Eleanor Morgan's *Anxiety for Beginners,* I have come to believe that fibromyalgia is another word for heightened anxiety in an extremely sensitive person; we do not discriminate information in our environment nor respond in the appropriate way. We live in constant apprehension of danger and our brains cannot monitor which stimuli is safe and which is dangerous.

What are the social implications of living with fibromyalgia? Telling someone about the condition is like speaking a foreign language. Most people are unclear about this dis-ease and their eyes cloud over when you tell them about it. The syndrome is difficult enough for the teller to describe, let alone the listener to understand. Inevitably they will ask if it is something like arthritis of the muscles, or an autoimmune disease. Even worse, they might label us as hypochondriacs.

Now shift for a moment and imagine telling someone you are a highly sensitive person. There is usually a little eyebrow lifting as the listener thinks one is being rather coy, attempting to shed a positive light on one's delicate self. But there is a difference if admitting you have a lot of anxiety.

Inevitably the person hearing this begins to tell you about medications or other strategies there are for this "psychological" problem. Of the above-mentioned terms, clearly, anxiety is the one which is more understandable by the general public.

These are among the many challenges of the chronically hyper-aroused fibromyalgia person. However, it is important to note that this syndrome is on a continuum and not all fit the same mold. Most of these personality traits began in childhood when the young person was usually considered shy and insecure. Perhaps they were genetic characteristics, or they became ultra sensitive early in life. They then developed anxiety, which in the words of Eleanor Morgan in *Anxiety for Beginners,* "involves excessive, unrealistic worry, avoidant behaviours and thoughts" (101).

Not everyone with anxiety has all of the same symptoms or traits or suffers to the same degree, but the similarities are quite astounding. Not all the hallmarks of anxiety and high sensitivity are negative either: who doesn't want to be intuitive and empathetic? Elaine Aron describes the traits of the highly sensitive person as a gift, while Scott Stossel suggests that anxiety can be seen as strength, resulting in a hard-working and diligent person.[2] So far few have written about the gifts or the strength of those of us suffering from fibromyalgia. Is it because this dis-ease is the end result of lifelong anxiety and hypersensitivity and is not actually a condition in and of itself? It would seem that the amygdala, the two nerve centers on either side of the thalamus in the brain that assess danger, is in overdrive, that is, it responds much more quickly to unexpected stimuli than that of most people.

I have read Stossel's book from cover to cover and I experienced a visceral response to his intense pain. Nonetheless, his scientific and historical analysis of anxiety is one which everyone with fibromyalgia should read, as his experience of anxiety is so similar to that of FMS. His inability to differentiate about whether or not anxiety is a "nurture or nature" phenomenon is one I have grappled with for decades regarding fibromyalgia. My small concern about the book is that he only briefly touches on the issue of neuroplasticity, the ability of the brain to change.

---

[2] See also Wendy Suzuki's *Good Anxiety: Harnessing the Power of the most Misunderstood Emotion.*

This now well-documented ability is the main cause for hope for those of us with anxiety or FMS.[3]

It is generally known that anxiety and depression generally go hand in hand. Anxiety involves negatively projecting the future while depression ruminates constantly upon the past. It would seem that both conditions are common among fibromyalgia (and PTSD sufferers). In the 2007 interview with Monica, she said, "I usually have a difficult time in the evening. Those are times when I feel more tired and probably more anxious and emotional. But, you know, sometimes I have it in the morning as well." Monica went on to say that sometimes she woke up feeling depressed. She also describes herself as someone who cares after others to the exclusion of caring for herself: "I don't usually take a lot of time out to take care of myself; just go and go, whatever someone else needed, regardless of how I felt. I've had a difficult time taking from anyone else or accepting help from others. I always just feel I'm taking advantage". Monica's words reflect the truth that we cannot take care of others if we can't take care of ourselves. We must practice self-compassion.

If we call ourselves highly sensitive, we can see benefits of our personal characteristics: we are intuitive, empathetic caregivers, hardworking, often creative and have the ability to thrive in spite of the challenges of everyday living. Through a non- judgmental acceptance of our strengths rather than fixating on our weaknesses there is hope for a better quality of life. Not all highly sensitive persons have fibromyalgia, nor do all highly anxious or depressed people have fibromyalgia symptoms.

We are highly sensitive people with rich and complex inner lives. We generally know a person's life history within minutes of meeting them. People easily confide in us, and we often take on their experiences and challenges. We suffer from sensory overload. We startle easily; we process sensory data differently than other people. Our nervous systems differ from those of the general population. We are highly empathetic and often intuitive beyond what is usual. Is it any wonder that our empathetic nervous systems react strongly to the pain we see in the world around us?

As mentioned earlier, anxiety-provoking thoughts reside in the amygdala, an area found in the midbrain which responds to threats,

---

[3] For more on neuroplasticity, see Norman Doidge's *The Brain that Changes Itself* and *The Brain's Way of Healing*.

causing us to be on high alert; staying in this zone for long periods of time leads to fatigue. For Monica, this fatigue was all too familiar: "I find it very difficult to do something as far as everyday living. I feel too tired to do something". Monica went on to discuss how she often felt guilty when she thought she was being lazy. She needed to be busy working, cleaning, and caring for her children, to her own detriment. She hated the perception of herself as lazy and did not want others to think that of her that way either. She was constantly fighting torpor.

Another interview participant from the 2007 book, Brenda, told this story of a visit to the doctor. After a doctor proclaimed her as looking healthy, he patted her on the head and "That was the end of it. So, it began a spiral of me saying 'Why do I feel this way? Why am I so tired?' And yet my vitality would come back, it was waxing and waning."

Whether or not the feeling that one must always be wary and "on duty" is a nature or nurture issue might seem irrelevant at this point, although in my view high degrees of anxiety in women is socially constructed. Given the societal expectations of women it is understandable that "hypervigilance" (a term I use frequently in my first book and one which Peter Levine discusses in Waking *the Tiger*) becomes overwhelming. The hypervigilant brain cannot distinguish between fear and flight, or rest and relaxation.

Unfortunately, fear and anxiety seem to accelerate as women with fibromyalgia grow older. It is likely that the same is true for men as well if they have not been able to heal the wounds and trauma of earlier times in their lives, or suffer from PTSD from their military service.

In a person who is extremely anxious, the brain cannot differentiate between a real or perceived threat. Indeed, there is a big difference between anxiety and fear, as discussed by the science writer Marantz Hening: "Anxiety is not fear, exactly, because fear is focused on something right in front of you, a real and objective danger. [Anxiety] is instead a kind of fear gone wild, a generalized sense of dread about something out there that seems menacing, but that in truth is not menacing, and may not even be out there." However, we can't reason anxiety away by admonishing ourselves that the worst will not ever happen, so the end result is the overwhelming fatigue that follows.

Fibromyalgia is quickly becoming an epidemic and living with the kinds of daily fear we all experience in a fast-paced, anxious world, worrying about justice inequities, homelessness, war and possibly catching Covid, it is likely to accelerate even more rapidly. I know anxiety and panic very well and it takes little to bring on a flare-up that I have to deal with along with chronic pain and fatigue. Feelings of peace are hard to come by. But life with fear being a constant in my life is not helpful for me or my loved ones. Instead, I <u>try</u> to exercise as much as I can, eat properly (except when chocolate is available!), sleep as much as I can, keep up with my friendships even if I'm tired, be productive as much as the fatigue will allow, and discipline myself to sit quietly and meditate for a few minutes each day. But more importantly, I try to be easy on myself and not feel guilty when I can't accomplish all these goals. I am no longer that high-achieving, rushing-about person I once was, and that's okay!

Fibromyalgia and Nurses

"Women never have a half-hour in all their lives (excepting
before or after anybody is up in the house) that they can call
their own, without fear of offending or of hurting someone."
– Florence Nightingale

In reviewing the extensive research I have conducted into FMS over the years, including interviews and blog comments, it has been interesting to observe that many of the commentators are nurses. This fits in with my view that it is caregivers who are predominantly women and highly sensitive, working in high-stress situations coupled with anxieties, who often say of their lives that they are burned out from a lifetime of caring for others. I continue to be amazed at how many nurses suffer from fibromyalgia brought on by a personal history of stress and anxiety, and usually precipitated by a crisis, an accident, surgery or something as seemingly simple as a root canal! In these days of Covid-19 we cannot help but speculate at the number of nurses who have developed (or will develop) fibromyalgia/PTSD/ chronic fatigue. We certainly know that nurses are burnt out; the news is full of stories regarding nurses leaving the profession. They are indeed heroines and heroes, but many have little energy to continue as caregivers.

One cannot speak of the nursing profession without mentioning Florence Nightingale. She was born of prominent British parents in Florence, Italy who were liberal-humanitarian social reformers. Her social activism led her to work during the Crimean War when England, France and the Ottoman Turks fought and won as allies against Russia. After the war, she came back to England with ideas on how to change the British army and hospitals, which she said needed good ventilation and whose sewers were considered defective. Lastly, she wanted properly trained nurses. It is because of her work and the book she wrote, the classic *Notes on Nursing,* that we can say that the nursing profession evolved.

From May 6-12th each year, we celebrate National Nurses' Week in honour of her birthday which was on May 12th, 1820. However, her birthday is now also celebrated as International Chronic Fatigue Syndrome and Fibromyalgia Awareness Day. It is now believed that Nightingale suffered from FMS and depression for most of her life.

Critics of Nightingale have speculated that she feigned illnesses, was bi-polar, and suffered from PTSD; these conditions were all due to various types of so-called hysteria, a term which demeans women and highly sensitive persons. My view is that she developed full-blown fibromyalgia after the trigger of contracting a fever in the Crimea while experiencing the horrific hospital, army and nursing conditions of war. But it is not as simple as that. For her to have developed fibromyalgia she needed the following personality and psychological characteristics: high sensitivity, and plagued with anxieties and past trauma. The war and finally a fever depleted her energy and her overwhelmed central nervous system. She could no longer work as effectively with the anxieties she had faced.

While the terms shell shock and PTSD seem to be different from fibromyalgia, they are from the same family. This fits with my view that fibromyalgia is socially induced in highly sensitive people (particularly women) whose central nervous system is in a state of chronic hyper-arousal. Dr. Kevin White calls fibromyalgia the "Nightingale Disease," and while I agree that many of the systems within the body eventually break down from this constant state of over stimulation of the CNS, I cannot agree with him that FMS is in and of itself an actual disease, rather a dis-ease. However, no one has yet to prove any particular theory about fibromyalgia, which is frustrating for both patients and health care providers. We can only continue to speculate, hoping for more concrete answers.

I refuse to think of Florence Nightingale as a malingerer considering all that she accomplished over her lifetime. She is like the many women I hear from daily who accomplish so much, caring for others, wanting to make an improvement in the lives of others while continuing to face their own challenges with pain and fatigue.

Famous FMS

"What I want for my fans and for the world, for anyone
who feels pain, is to lean into that pain and embrace it as
much as they can and begin the healing process."
– Lady Gaga

A few months ago, I learned that Lady Gaga was hospitalized and had cancelled performances because of fibromyalgia. Those of us who share her condition can especially commiserate with her during what must have been a severe flare-up. More troubling is the fact that the kind of high stress profession she is involved with does not allow much time for rest.

There has rarely been so much public awareness of fibromyalgia as there is now that Lady Gaga has become public about her own suffering. I know little about Lady Gaga and wonder why it takes a widely-known singer/ performer to convince some members of the public to take fibromyalgia seriously.

I have been researching historical figures who have been deemed hypochondriac because of the vague ailments and symptoms which mimic fibromyalgia. Along with Florence Nightingale, the classical composer Robert Schumann was said to be highly sensitive as a young man and suffered greatly at age 16 after his father and brother died. Canadian pianist Glenn Gould was also said to be someone who was a "malingerer," a common derogatory word that is used to describe those with invisible pain conditions. He suffered from pains and was a worrier. Charles Darwin was a very anxious person and had pains and fatigue. The list is long. We with FMS are in the company of many brilliant, talented people!

In more recent years, celebrities like Morgan Freeman and singer Sinead O'Connor have revealed that they, too, suffer from fibromyalgia. O'Connor's words about her condition are telling: "When you get something like fibromyalgia it's a gift, actually, because you have to reassess your life." But I personally do not consider it a gift!

Symptoms of FMS: An Introduction

In this section, I explore and compare the symptoms of fibromyalgia from my own experiences and the research I have undertaken over the years. Their numbers are vast. Some are the result of fibromyalgia while others are not specifically related to the syndrome; as mentioned, it is often difficult to differentiate. They include

sleep disturbances
nightmares and night terrors
enhanced startle reflex
sensitivities to weather changes
light sensitivity
panic attacks
social anxiety

Physical symptoms include

muscular pain
itching
tingling in the arms and hands
restless legs
shortness of breath
red or pinkish palms
gastric distress

Additional debilitating symptoms include

> depression
> phobias
> hypervigilance
> fatigue
> fainting
> sensitivity to noise, excitement, and strong smells
> chemical sensitivities
> carpal tunnel syndrome
> intolerance to vigorous exercise

Anxious persons with highly sensitive personalities are often easily overwhelmed, cautious, overly reflective, sometimes have low self esteem, and are greatly concerned about health. Often, they are highly intuitive, easily over stimulated, prone to catastrophic thinking, constant worriers, and apprehensive. They are usually highly motivated and "on the go" mentally and physically, although as FMS symptoms become worse, low energy ensues.

Those of us with FMS have been called jumpy, neurotic, malingers, and high strung, among other names that stigmatize. Speaking of her unwillingness to be in the doctor's office very often, Monica said her fear was he would think she was a hypochondriac. However, it is fear that is behind all of this; fear which is often unspoken. Taken all together, these symptoms affect our perceptions of ourselves as high maintenance and make us feel incapable of managing our own lives. They act as talismans that link us to our past. They are the physical representation of our life's journey. Not all of us have all of the above symptoms and many are transient. Given that many are symptomatic of other life-threatening diseases it is little wonder that fear of each of them can induce catastrophic thinking.

I have found that while the symptoms of FMS are generally agreed upon, it is not so easily accepted that anxiety is at the root of the syndrome. Because we are so susceptible to the symptoms mentioned, I am hesitant to record those which are the most common, which is why support groups which discuss mainly symptoms but do not address the cause can be counter-productive. Nonetheless all the symptoms can be viewed as interconnected.

It appears that most of us suffering from chronic ailments need the support of others who are also challenged by the same symptoms. While I originally thought that the pain and chronic fatigue would be the most common, I was amazed to find that, in fact, it was my blog posts on itching and pins and needles which received the most daily reading and comments from others around the world. In my view pain and chronic fatigue are the most debilitating of the symptoms and what define fibromyalgia, while other symptoms are off shoots that arise from an overstimulated central nervous system.

Itching

"The itch sensation is a perception."
– Dr. Zhou-Feng Chen

What could possibly be happening to the person with fibromyalgia who cannot find relief from itching so severe that it causes open wounds? Unlike the frustrations of a disease such as eczema, a fungal infection, or an autoimmune disorder like psoriasis, the itching of fibromyalgia does not seem to have a specific label which can be attached to it.

Responses to my blog postings reveal that this is one of the most common complaints about living with fibromyalgia, though there are many who do not experience these debilitating bouts of itching. Itching can occur at any time and can be brought about by many factors. For many, it is a weather change or a cold, humid or hot spell. For others, itching can occur after a stressful or exciting occasion. We have to become sleuths and try to document when itching is at its worst.

Let's begin by considering the location of the itching: our skin. Skin is meant to protect us and is always renewing itself. It is not meant to be a source of irritation to our psyches. Touch is one of our lovely senses, and skin is where we experience touch. Think of the soothing words that can be associated with skin: "soft as a baby's skin," "soft to the touch," "skin as smooth as silk," "soft as a mother's touch" and so many more that evoke a feeling of love and tenderness. But there are many cases when the skin itself can become our own enemy.

The skin is the largest organ of the body with more than 4 million receptors which help to identify stimuli like pressure, heat, cold and pain. When one of the sensory receptors is stimulated there is an electrical signal that is taken to a nerve cell that carries nerve impulses to the central nervous system (CNS). The CNS responds through the motor neurons, a nerve cell that carries messages from the brain and spinal cord to stimulate or contract muscles. The muscles and glands interpret the messages and will either contract or relax. It seems likely that in fibromyalgia there is a disruption in the neurotransmitters and intense itching occurs in particular when there are unusual events that the brain interprets as unfamiliar. Often, for me, it is when the weather changes, particularly on rainy, humid or windy days, that I feel the need to scratch. The itching is usually, but not exclusively, most severe in my hands and feet, although it can often feel like it is all over my body.

The itch sensation (its medical name is pruritus) is caused by a subset of what is known as C-fibers, classified as pain-fibers (or nociceptors). There is an overlap between itch and pain neurons; therefore, because those of us with fibromyalgia have pain, the same neurological systems are activated. The itch neurons are in the peripheral nervous system (PNS) just outside the central nervous system (CNS). In other words, neuropathic pain that we experience often causes neuropathic itch. It is the least understood among the somatic senses. While neuropathic pain is more frequent on the face, head and neck, the many comments I have had from readers of my blogs have complained about itching in both the upper and the lower extremities. This syndrome is called "polyneuropathies." This itching is usually worse in hot weather and subsides somewhat in cold, and yet rapid changes in temperature can also affect itching. Treatment for itching is not easy as those with fibromyalgia pain taking opioid pain relievers will find the itching becomes worse. Furthermore, neuropathic pain does not respond well to antihistamines.

There are many terms for chronic itching: "neuropathic itch (NI)," "pruritus," "distressing sensory symptoms," "self- injurious scratching," and even "phantom itching" are terms that are often used inter-changeably. I prefer NI for fibromyalgia itch as it reflects the origin of the disorder in the nervous system.

In an effort to understand the source of FMS-related itching, I have undertaken some research; in an article entitled "The Itch," American surgeon and writer Atul Gawande discusses the psychological link with physical itching:

> We experience things that seem physically real but aren't: sensations of itching that arise from nothing more than itchy thoughts; dreams that can seem indistinguishable from reality; phantom sensations that amputees have in their missing limbs. [The itching we experience in fibromyalgia is "phantom itching."] The more we examine the actual nerve transmissions we receive from the world outside, the more inadequate they seem.[4]

It seems that the brain takes on a variety of signals to recreate sensory experiences from our past, but the question arises about how we can retrain our brain to become less hypersensitive? I refer the reader to the work of Diane Jacobs PT who uses a technique called "dermoneuromodulation" to help calm the central and peripheral nervous system. Though not an easy read, it may be helpful (https://www.dermoneuromodulation.com/)

Further ground-breaking research regarding itching comes from professor Dr. Zhou-Feng Chen and his colleagues at the Washington University School of Medicine Pain Center where he serves as the director of the Center for the Study of Itch. To quote from his biography: "Ongoing research… is centered on signalling and synaptic mechanisms of itch transmission from skin to the brain and crosstalk between itch and pain." While it appears that the team has focussed its research primarily on mice, the avenue is hopeful for those of us with chronic pain and itching and its link to brain activity. I recommend a visit to Dr. Chen's website to keep up to date on his team's research: https://itch.wustl.edu/.

Jacobs and Gawande both indicate that itching is related to the perception or rather, misperception of the brain which must be retrained. Even reading about itching can cause us to want to scratch!

Retraining the brain is an answer for itching. But that takes an awfully long time and in an acute attack is not very helpful, nor are many of us aware how to do this. In the meantime, cold packs help somewhat as does meditation and other relaxing practices to soothe the nervous system before the itching happens. You can try massaging the affected area gently when the itching begins or relax using CBD oil (see section on cannabis). Hypoallergenic moisture creams can be somewhat useful, as can noticing

---

[4] The New Yorker Annals of Medicine, 8/27/2008

when the last attack happened and under what conditions so that we can avoid triggers. For me, this is about watching the weather reports and trying to find ways of calming my nervous system when I know a dramatic weather change is about to happen. This is difficult as I live in a climate where weather changes rapidly much of the year!

What else can be done to help the itch? I urge readers to practice a daily relaxation strategy, practice box breathing, exercise in moderation, undertake a hobby that is new to you, as well as creative and repetitive, and most importantly, work towards decreasing stimuli to the nervous system. **Be sure that you have been thoroughly checked out by a medical professional to determine that it is indeed a neuropathic itch due to fibromyalgia.**

In my own case, perhaps because I am taking a low dose of Gabapentin, a medication used to control nerve pain, I seem to have less itching than my readers. Research suggests that this medication is somewhat effective for some and I believe it is for me. (Note: I now only take 100 mgs of Gabapentin at night and since this is the lowest dose there is, it probably is not very effective with chronic itching.)

Numbness and Pins and Needles

"The world is full of suffering; it is also full of overcoming it."
– Helen Keller

Those of us with fibromyalgia have what is known as **peripheral neuropathy**, that is, pain mostly in the legs, tingling of the extremities, pins and needles, numbness, and "falling asleep" of legs or arms. For me it is much worse at night and centred in my arms rather than my legs. The result is that I wake up several times during the night when an arm is "asleep," numb with cold and actually hurting. When I am up for awhile, moving about, the feeling comes back in my arm and I fall back asleep only to wake up an hour or two later with numbness on the other side. My sleep is very disturbed by this relatively new symptom that is quite common among those of us with FMS.

Unlike diabetics who often have these symptoms constantly, those of us with FMS usually experience them during a flare-up. When this occurs, it is time to stop, take stock of what is happening in our minds, and work with our pain rather than struggle against it. Not an easy job!

I was very sleep deprived during a flare-up yet I dread going to bed knowing that a few hours later I would awaken with hurting arms. I still do all the suggested right things: Epsom salts bath before going to bed and applying heat to my neck during the day. I put a small pillow under my neck to support the area that is not on a pillow, and I have the right pillow for my upper body. I try to discipline myself to meditate each day and I also do some gentle movements of my arms often during the day. One particular stretch which does help somewhat is standing against the wall with my arms outstretched against the wall and my head against the surface with a forward look, but not jutting my chin outward, for one minute.

Movement is said to be good for tingling, numbness and pins and needles sensations. Yet, in spite of all my good intentions, the demon often persists. It is difficult to maintain a positive outlook with such constant disruption of sleep.

I recently had the nerve conduction test that evaluates the function and conduction of the motor and sensory nerves of the body, and it was determined that I have carpal tunnel syndrome. I have now had carpal tunnel surgery on both hands and while the numbness has disappeared, my hands continue to ache.

In the following sections I discuss the senses and how they are all connected to one another and often affected by the malfunctioning central nervous system.

Painful teary eyes

"Of all the senses, sight must be the most delightful."
– Helen Keller

Two years ago, I had a dreadful pain in my eye. I rushed to the eye doctor who did many tests and could not find anything wrong with it. The next day it was gone. This week, it came back and I had an "aha moment." Maybe it is a fibro flare-up! This time the pain lasted all day, even with using the over-the-counter drops. It was as though someone was sticking something in my eye.

I did some research and discovered that many people have intense pain in the eyes. More women than men suffer from cataracts and dry eyes, according to the Harvard Health Publishing Medical School booklet. I have had both cataract surgeries and dry eyes. Dry eyes are a most annoying condition as it looks as though I am crying, but not all people who have watery eyes have fibromyalgia.

I have had teary eyes in the past, to my embarrassment. The itching in the eyes is almost as dreadful as the pain and crying. In addition, I am photosensitive; I cannot tolerate bright light. I am fairly certain there is a relationship of eye problems to fibromyalgia, and I am sorry that the eye doctor did not pick that up! I think we need a label on our foreheads to tell the world that we are unique and please treat us accordingly. After all, if I have had itching in other places, why is it different if it affects the eyes as well as the skin?

Along with dry eyes (known as "sicca syndrome" and also affecting the nose and mouth) certain patterns of light can affect our eyes which arise from stimuli such as trees swaying or fast-moving scenes in a movie.

There are many external conditions that affect our eyes: overhead fluorescent lights, or windy days outside without sunglasses, the glare of snow, flashing lights in a TV program. Light sensitivity is also a symptom associated with concussion (or mild traumatic brain injury); wearing sunglasses, even indoors, can help to reduce the glare from a too-bright world.

What's that smell?

"For the sense of smell, almost more than any other, has the power
to recall memories and it is a pity that we use it so little."
– Rachel Carson

Imagine a rose and the strong scent it evokes. What is the brain's reaction? Hopefully it is a joyous one. However, for some this aroma might be troublesome as it could be associated with a tragic or unhappy event. A good smell for some may be a bad one for others. As an example, for me the smell of popcorn in a movie theatre makes me nauseous, although I do not have bad memories of movie theatres or popcorn, which I quite like! Going into a home where wood is burning makes me cough and there is increasing evidence that home wood stoves and fireplaces are unhealthy, although not everyone reacts overtly to that smell and many love the smell of burning wood in a home fireplace or stove. What are we to make of this other than we with this syndrome of fibromyalgia often have a hypersensitive nose?

These neurological dysfunctions and contradictions of ours often cannot be fully understood. It is easy to comprehend how the chemicals from the perfume or soap aisle in a department store or pharmacy can cause many of us to feel dizzy, nauseated, lightheaded, and short of breath. Many of us react badly to the smell of aftershave, or any perfumes and cologne but love the scent of the natural oils of lavender, patchouli or sandalwood. Hair spray or strong shampoos can bring about a feeling of weakness and walking in a shop that does cosmetic nails or some hair salons can be overwhelming. This reaction can be the body reacting to triggers which may or may not have associations with our past. But it may also be a CNS reaction within our bodies responding to extreme stimuli.

This is the case of Multiple Chemical Sensitivities (MCS), a twin to fibromyalgia, from buildings which are considered "sick buildings" and in which people develop sensitivities from toxic substances.

One of the women I interviewed, Monica, reported that "the smell of things like contact cement and things like that... makes me very sick. Quite often I'll lose my voice. I have headaches. I have difficulty breathing, tightness in my chest." It is fortunate that many government offices, schools, and hospitals have adopted scent-free policies.

Deb, another woman I interviewed, had multiple chemical sensitivities, multiple sclerosis, and fibromyalgia that were almost certainly related to workplace exposure to toxic substances. She worked in a textile mill: "My office was very, very damp and there was no insulation, just a concrete block on the outside of the wall. Within a year my window had turned black from mould. I worked from 6 a.m. till 6 p.m. and then my system couldn't handle anymore. This was the beginning of how I got sick, that's where my allergies developed, and I became allergic to everything."

I never did work in an office of the kind that Deb had to work in; I had a large window which would bring in lovely clear air. Have I inherited my sensitivity from a mother who responded in a panic to loud noises and strong odours and would ask repeatedly, "What IS that smell?" Like my mother, I can tell immediately if a person has been in a place where food has been cooking, and like my mother, this smell on someone's clothing can make me feel nauseous. I believe my sensitivity to smell may be somewhat typical of those with FMS.

A small study conducted in Tel-Aviv University with fibromyalgia volunteers, however, suggests a different story. The research took place in 2014 with 24 people who had FMS, a control group and another group of sclerosis patients. The study published in *Immunologic Research* ("Olfactory impairment in patients with fibromyalgia syndrome and systemic sclerosis") suggests the fibromyalgia sample had the worst sense of smell of all the groups and it impacted on taste. They used Sniffin' Sticks as their "instrument" for testing smell (these tests allow an assessment of a patient's olfactory performance). Since this is a very small sample it cannot be used as proof that the sense of smell is decreased in patients with fibromyalgia. The jury is still out! Many of us do lose some of our hearing and have no sense of smell or taste. Still others cannot bear to be touched and many, many more of us are sensitive to light, perfumes, after shave lotion and temperature changes. It is up to us individually to keep tabs on that which causes discomfort to our senses.

These words of Sir William Osler (1849–1919), a Canadian physician and educator, may serve to guide us in our observations: "Observe, record, tabulate, communicate. Use your five senses…learn to see, listen to hear, learn to feel, learn to *smell* [my italics] and know that by practice alone you can become expert." While he may have been writing this to his fellow physicians, those of us with FMS have to become the medical experts of our own lives.

The Inner Ear: Dizziness and Vertigo

"The ear is the avenue to the heart."
– Voltaire

Just as I thought I had experienced everything unusual with regard to this frustrating dis-ease, fibromyalgia, I developed another aggravating symptom: vertigo. It began at night; when I turned over in bed, the room began spinning. This episode was very frightening and lasted about 30 seconds, followed by nausea. I had another episode the next night as well. The morning after the second episode, leaning forward, I had a very violent attack which prompted me to go to the doctor.

This vertigo is not to be confused with the kind of dizziness that is brief and passes quickly. Rather, benign paroxysmal positional vertigo (or BPPV), as it is known, is experienced as spinning. In BPPV, small calcium crystals become lodged in the inner ear, causing malaise, but they can be encouraged to move through by a technique called the Epley manoeuvre. The doctor asked me if I was game to try this technique and I agreed. Lying on the table my head was hanging somewhat over the end while he held my head and rotated it for 30 seconds. This manoeuvre is described on the Mayo Clinic website and it is suggested that the person can try this at home.

I can attest to it being one of the worst experiences I have had in many years. The doctor did this to my head three times, both sides, and the nausea and dizziness became unbearable, resulting in the need for a nurse to administer a Gravol injection. Obviously, the manoeuvre did not work.

A few weeks went by and on the advice of friends I made an appointment with a physiotherapist who specializes in vestibular issues, among them vertigo. He spent an hour and a half testing me; while I was wearing a specialized face mask with wires attached to a computer, he watched my eye movements on the computer (after he had determined which ear and where in the ear the crystals were located) then we proceeded with the treatment which was much gentler than the previous one, causing only mild dizziness. I had been shaking beforehand fearing the worst, but soon relaxed as I realized he knew what he was doing. I was told to take it easy for the rest of the day and to keep my head still, neither looking up nor down and sleeping on my back that night. The following day I was to test the vertigo and luckily for me this one treatment worked. He had told me that there was an 85% chance it would work after the first visit and if a second was needed, it would rise to a 95% success rate.

I smile now remembering waking up without fear of the room spinning. This physio is amazing in that he knows so much about FMS and migraines (which he believes are similar in that they are the result of people who have different "brain wiring" than most others). For that reason, he handles fibromyalgia patients with great sensitivity and understanding, given our own sensitivities. I am so lucky to have found him. I have now learned that physiotherapists (called physical therapists in the US) are taught how to treat vertigo in school. Seven years later after another attack, I quickly repeated the process. The crystals this time were located in the front canal, different than the first time where they were in the middle of the three canals. Again, one manoeuvre and the vertigo disappeared.

Unfortunately, vertigo is only one of several ear-related problems I have experienced. My ears often crackle, feel like they are submerged in water, feel full, itch, flutter and sometimes just feel odd. My hearing is not good, particularly on certain days. Finally, as suggested by a hearing specialist who works with FMS, I succumbed to hearing aids. However, they are not comfortable as my ears feel attacked by this encumbrance, so I only wear them while watching television.

Hearing loss appears to be common after a prolonged history of fibromyalgia.

It seems as though *sensorineural hearing loss*, that is, loss that is due to damage to the inner ear auditory nerve pathways to the brain, occurs more frequently in those with fibromyalgia than has been reported. Not hearing lovely sounds like music can have devastating effects on a person's morale. It stands to reason that the tension and anxiety that goes hand

and hand with fibromyalgia would result in jaw clenching, teeth grinding and tightened neck muscles, thereby affecting, among other muscles and nerves, the seventh cranial nerve which supplies all the muscles of the face.

In connection with hearing issues, many have written to ask me if TMJ (temporomandibular disorder) is common with fibromyalgia. TMJ is the result of the twisting of the jaw joint that slides and rotates just in front of the ear and happens during the opening or closing of the mouth, or side motion movements. Some telltale signs of TMJ: sensitive teeth (no doubt because so many of us have unexplained tooth pain) and earaches. The jaw muscles refer the pain to the teeth and ears and can even cause headaches.

The main nerve for the jaw joint is attached to the TMJ disk so that when it is compressed it tightens nerve and blood vessels around the ear and temples, especially if one has stiff neck muscles. Sometimes ringing in the ears (tinnitus) is a common complaint as well.

Often background noise and/or many people talking in a room results in great sensitivity to noise in people with this type of hearing loss.

This is just one more challenge for those of us who grind our teeth, absorb tension in our necks and jaws and suffer from headaches and earaches. Another reason for us to educate our health care professionals and especially our dentists and dental assistants that fibromyalgia does not leave a nerve in our bodies in peace! Furthermore, hearing loss impacts on our daily lives and our personal relationships. Hopefully we will *hear* more about the complexity of hearing loss and fibromyalgia in the near future.

Noise Sensitivity

"One of the greatest sounds of them all—and to me
it is a sound—is utter, complete silence."
– Andre Kostelanetz

The term "misophonia" refers to sounds which can cause severe reactions in certain people. Many of us with fibromyalgia experience extreme discomfort over certain sounds. For me it is the clicking of heels on pavement, a dog slurping its food, chewing loudly by others, the humming of a motor or heating system, a baby crying, boom boxes...the list is endless. Even more alarming is an unexpected loud noise, such as a motorcycle or firecrackers. I realize that most people can find many of these sounds alarming, but for the person with noise sensitivity, the auditory nervous system is in overdrive. The startle reflex can easily click in.

Dr. Sonia Lupien and her colleagues at the University of Montreal are doing research on the "larger amygdala." My suspicion is that those of us with fibromyalgia have an unusually large amygdala which scans for threats in the environment to the extent that many sounds evoke stress or emotionally upsetting episodes.

Noise sensitivity appear to have a genetic component; in my family, my father often complained about certain noises or sounds that did not seem to affect anyone else. According to Dr. Aage Moller, a neuroscientist at the University of Texas who specializes in the auditory nervous system, noise sensitivity is "hard-wired, like right or left-handedness and is probably not an auditory disorder but a 'physiological abnormality' that resides in brain structures activated by processed sound."[5]

---

[5] Mollet quoted in Joyce Cohen, "Misophonia", *The Globe and Mail*, Sept. 7, 2001.

While research into sound sensitivity so far has not discovered an effective treatment for this condition, I believe we **can** create new neural pathways that would allow us over time to deal more effectively with misophonia.

My suggestion is to fill the day with lovely sounds that bring about joy instead of irrational fear: listen to your favourite music and to people who have soothing voices, or the sound of rippling water in a stream, soft laughter and other pleasing experiences that soothe the ears. Not always easy, and I still cross the street if I hear the clickety clack of high heels on the pavement!

Tooth Pain

"If your teeth are clenched and your fists are
clenched, your lifespan is probably clenched."
– Adabella Radici

I once experienced my first toothache. It happened out of the blue, a
bottom front tooth that had never been decayed, nor capped. The pain
was excruciating and unrelenting. Being 4000 miles away from home, in
a hotel on another coast, the pain was even more disturbing. I quickly
searched out a dentist nearby and found a young, knowledgeable dentist
who was very calming. X-rays revealed no abscesses or cavities and the
gums were in good condition. She speculated that it might be due to
fibromyalgia and indeed it was.

Like many with FMS, I tend to focus on the "biggie" symptoms:
pain, fatigue, depression and sleep disorders. We may become so used
to these familiar symptoms that we forget how patterns can sometimes
shift, and new symptoms can appear. With FMS, rarely are two days
alike. Tooth pain is new for me, though pain in others parts of my body
is sadly commonplace. Why my teeth? I have had facial pain in the past,
shock-like, jabbing pains that were somewhat transient. But this horrific
pain was something new.

Could the pain be related to new trigger points caused by clenching my
jaw and grinding my teeth at night, I wondered? Does the nervous system
never take a rest? Could the pain be related to a difficult root canal just
a month ago on a molar on the other side of my mouth? I remember that
the muscles in my jaws became so tight! Now the new tooth pain began to

fit. Trigger points shift often. Why did I think my teeth would be exempt? Will this last, I wondered? Will the muscles in my neck and jaws relax and the pain shift to another locale? Just one more question of many in living with the demon of fibromyalgia.

Neuropathic Pain

"Pain is real when you get other people to believe in it."
– Naomi Wolf

There are two kinds of pain: nociceptive and neuropathic. Nociceptive pain occurs as the result of a harmful action like a cut or burn, or from surgery. It is usually temporary. Those of us with fibromyalgia suffer from the more complex and challenging neuropathic pain, which is the result of long-term damage to the nervous system that has become chronic. Opioids offer only temporary relief. Many find some degree of relief from their pain with Gabapentin or Pregabalin.

Neuropathic pain is complicated, and though some with FMS resort to taking them, highly addictive opioids are not the answer. While I advocate for mild exercise as one form of self-help, sometimes more strenuous activity is warranted. Many of us can hardly tolerate any exercise at all, mild or vigorous. Strenuous activity usually brings about fibro flare-ups (I found this out with increasing activity and stretching following hip replacement surgery in order to help with walking and avoiding limping). Now I am in a quandary as to how much to do without increasing my pain level. My brain keeps me travelling down that same old painful neural pathway. Training the brain is not an easy task, but there is little option. Mindfulness, meditation, breathing exercises, walking in spite of pain, exercise like biking on my recumbent bike, are my strategies, and I have an understanding chiropractor who tells me I expect too much of myself. I need to remind myself that being hard on ourselves is a hallmark of those with fibromyalgia.

I cannot overstate how complex daily living becomes for those of us with neuropathic pain. We have to be kind to ourselves and recognize that self-compassion is key to our quality of life.

Neuropathy can occur in many parts of the body; for me, the legs are an area where I experience neuropathy's characteristic muscle weakness and pain. This makes me fearful of re-exacerbating the pain by exercising, yet inactivity is also a trigger for pain. While neuropathy is common in such conditions as diabetes, people with fibromyalgia experience the same symptoms, which are pain, tingling, pins and needles, and weakness. I have these symptoms in both legs and arms as well as sharp shooting pains often in my back and shoulders. I have to confess that Gabapentin does help with painful episodes. Unfortunately, the side effects of weight gain and groggy head are very frustrating.

There are many who believe that reducing the anxiety that comes with painful episodes is more effective than dealing with the pain directly. But if one has lived with severe chronic pain for most of her adult life, changing the brain is not an easy task. To add to all this, my body is now chronically unconditioned. I don't move in a way that brings about good balance and posture. My muscles have weakened, and I need frequent massages, physiotherapy and chiropractic treatments. The question always arises: will I ever walk in comfort again as I did just few short years ago?

Foot Pain

"When things get really bad, just raise your glass
and stamp your feet and do a little jig."
– Leonard Cohen

I began to have foot pain after my hip surgery, a condition I had never had before. I speculated about the cause: Too little walking? Plantar fasciitis? Shifting from soft sponge shoes to sneakers which are heavier? Shuffling after the surgery? The possibilities were endless. No one has been able to tell me what it is that inhibits my walking and causes almost shock-like pain in the arches and the top of the foot.

Once more I was in a quandary and began thinking the foot pain was just a fibromyalgia symptom. Why not? The dis-ease affects all my muscles, joints and body parts so why would my feet be immune? Of course, this is a dangerous state of mind. One can have other conditions that cannot be blamed on fibromyalgia. But the puzzle about my feet persisted. Should I try other shoes? It is important for everyone to have good shoes without high heels and good arch support, whether or not we have fibromyalgia.

Sometimes, the reason for my foot pain is clear, like when I wear something other than the sensible shoes that are my daily companions. This time, I did not wear high heels, (in fact, I don't own any), but the shoes were admittedly a bit dressier than my usual funky coloured sneakers. Given that my muscles have become weakened over the years because of my inability to sustain regular exercise due to FMS, I have found that supportive shoes are the best answer to stability. For that reason, I decided to brighten my days with coloured sneakers that also bring a smile to others. But without them, my legs and feet are painful, especially at night.

I have been having reflexology treatments for my feet, which are very soothing and comforting while they last, though their effects disappear quickly. Foot massages are lovely and I do them myself. Massages are paramount as is all touch. Despite all my efforts, pain in the arches and tops of feet persist, and my research on fibromyalgia and foot pain did not yield any answers.

Because I suffer from low back pain caused by bulging discs, I was referred to a chronic pain clinic where I met with a wonderful registered nurse and a phenomenal physician who explained degenerative disc disease and lumbar spine pain. I learned about pain from these discs which can radiate down the legs and feet. Aging is not for cowards! One thing leads to another, and it is a matter of joining together the dots of the body's complex, yet wonderful central nervous system and its relationship to the brain, which extends to the feet.

The staff at the pain clinic told me that the majority of their clients have fibromyalgia. When I gave the physician my short version of fibromyalgia, he said it was "well stated"[6].

So, what about my sore feet now that it is established that my spine, which has normal age-related disc degeneration, is sending messages to my brain that walking hurts my feet?

There is some degree of help available through paravertebral nerve blocks (a form of temporary anesthetic a bit like an epidural) which may temporarily help with leg and foot pain, but I was advised that fibromyalgia clients do not do as well as others with disc disease, as our pain originates from chronic central nervous system overstimulation. Nonetheless, I am happy there is the possibility I will be walking for longer periods of time without foot and back pain!

One effective treatment I have discovered for foot pain is pool walking, which removes pressure from the joints and the feet. Regular walking for short periods of time (15 minutes) several times a day is also helpful, as is walking with trekking sticks.

---

[6] I recommend this website for those with chronic foot pain: https://healthskills. wordpress.com/if-you-have-chronic-pain/

As cannabis is now legal in Canada, I have found a very good CBD ointment which has been helpful for pain and especially for foot pain. If you live in a jurisdiction where cannabis products are still not legal, ask your doctor about obtaining a medical exemption.

Spasms and Restless Legs

"Am I alone in my egotism when I say that never does the pale
light of dawn filter through the blinds of 52 Tavistock Square but
I open my eyes and exclaim 'Good God! Here I am again,' not
always with pleasure, often with pain, sometimes in a spasm."
– Virginia Woolf

The body of someone suffering from fibromyalgia is often very sensitive
to even gentle touch without experiencing pain. Muscles are tense, often
in spasm, aching, and after prolonged use can become even more stressed.
Exercise, the mantra of those who want to become or remain fit, often
creates more pain for those of us with FMS, unless it is very gentle. Even
then, for some, *any* kind of movement can precipitate episodes of severe
pain. What are people to do who cannot exercise, move, even walk slowly
without wondering which body parts will break out in agony? The younger
person begins to feel even older, and the older person is additionally
burdened with the aches and pains of aging.

There are distinct kinds of severe muscle responses to exercise, the most
common being agonizing spasms, accompanied by the nervous system's
restless legs and trapped nerves that together can play havoc for the FMS
person contemplating exercise of any kind.

Spasms, often referred to as charley horses, can be excruciating and
numerous. One of the women I interviewed for the first book told me she
often has them non-stop at night accompanied by restless legs, and both
prevent her from restorative sleep. She gets relief only by heavy medications
and long soaks in the bath.

What is it about exercise that brings about more pain for the FMS
sufferer? The pain may be caused by an overstimulation of the adrenal

glands, leading to adrenal fatigue or exhaustion. The adrenals are small glands located on top of each kidney. One of the important hormones that they produce is cortisol, which helps with counteracting inflammation in the muscles. They also produce adrenaline, which we feel in a rush when we exercise.

We are (or were before fibromyalgia) high energy people with extreme empathy and deep emotional responses. The result of these qualities is that the adrenals are on high alert, producing more and more adrenaline and cortisol when we are in fight or flight mode. The result of this excess of cortisol is loss of sleep, inability to "shut off," muscle pain, fatigue, carpal tunnel syndrome, weakness, and depression.

Extreme sensitivity of our muscles results in both chronic and acute pain. One of the women I interviewed, Marg, said that pain in her hands was brought on by even simple actions like peeling vegetables. Several other the women had carpal tunnel syndrome, as I did. It's little wonder that expending extra energy through exercise throws our normal daily rhythm of cortisol balancing even further out of whack.

Most exercise requires the use of the legs. However, because the debilitating neurological disorder called restless leg syndrome (RLS) is so common among people with FMS, the added burden of increased movement of the legs can result in increased severity of symptoms of RLS. The sensations with this syndrome are peculiar and words as *burning, creepy, crawly,* or *uncomfortable* do not adequately describe them. One constantly has the urge to move about and lying flat in bed at night is probably the worst time of all. Add to this the extra energy used during exercise and one can see that an already overextended nervous system will increase the discomfort and often painful RLS since it is likely that the hyper-arousal will not subside easily.

The muscles of the fibromyalgia sufferer are tight and often contracted. They may have become shortened, or perhaps conversely overextended from stretching too vigorously, resulting in decreased mobility. As a result of contractions due to pain, it is little wonder that nerves become "trapped" in various locations throughout the body. While little has been written about this, I believe that this occurs more frequently than has been reported. Constant excruciating pain in specific parts of the body that are very localized are often perplexing, but I suspect not uncommon. My own trapped nerve is located just below one knee, bringing numbness to an area about the size of a small pancake. I have found that the best relief for pain is slow motion, walking or pool walking for short periods of time. Walking for extended periods of time or walking rapidly exacerbates pain in other parts of the body.

Along with slow, deliberate movement, deep breathing and strengthening exercises are most helpful for quieting the nervous system along with increasing mobility. As mentioned previously, vigorous activity and stretching is to be avoided.

Brain Fog

"My own brain is to me the most unaccountable of
machinery—always buzzing, humming, soaring,
roaring, diving, and then buried in mud."
– Virginia Woolf

To live a life in a state of high anxiety bordering on panic is common among those of us with fibromyalgia. It seems as though our brains are hardwired for worry and then worrying about worrying. We anticipate pain, fatigue, muddled thoughts, and a myriad of other symptoms almost every waking (and sleeping!) hour. It has become a habit that often seems unbreakable and depression and fear set in. Accompanying these is brain fog, the confusion that often does not allow us to focus or to think clearly. Some describe the sensation as "fuzzy brain," "spaced out," "dreamy," "brain farts," or just plain forgetfulness. Whatever the label, those of us with the condition know it is often accelerated by over stimulation, but especially by lack of sleep. The medical term for brain fog is *dyscognition*.

The statistics regarding the self-described symptoms of fibromyalgia, including brain fog, are staggering. They range from 10% to 15% of the population, while it is suspected that the numbers of unreported cases are even higher. It is likely that numbers will soar as more military personnel are open to discussing the agonizing effects of post-traumatic stress disorder (PTSD). When I read the symptoms reported by veterans, most of whom are diagnosed with PTSD, I immediately recognize what we have described as fibromyalgia. Somehow, though, the label of PTSD seems to be more acceptable to the experts than fibromyalgia. Nevertheless, in my view they are identical twins and changing the names and labels is not particularly useful. Certainly, however, dyscognition is common among those of us with PTSD and fibromyalgia, particularly when over-stimulated.

The brain is about three pounds and sometimes it feels like 100 to those of us who are constantly in a buzzed state. It would seem that the brain has difficulty in responding to stimuli because of a hyper-aroused central nervous system, a phrase I keep repeating over and over again. These habits of the brain are strong and require discipline that is challenging to break free from since they have accumulated over many years. Stress and all that it encompasses is one of the main culprits, along with too much sitting and especially during recent times, too much isolation during Covid. Under these conditions, we are easy prey to anxiety and despair.

Generally, our brain fog becomes worse when we are multi-tasking. When we begin to try to complete many tasks at the same time, our overworked central nervous system rebels and we become overwhelmed. Women are generally the gender which suffers the most from attempts to multitask, I believe.

When we reach the depths of despair believing that there is no hope, we *can* change our approach to our challenges. It does require effort, but we and we alone can do it. The difficulty comes in old age when there is generalized forgetfulness and brain fog becomes more common. Other times of reported increased brain fog can occur during pregnancy and menopause.

Along with the disciplined practice of mindfulness meditation (discussed in depth in a subsequent section) is that of movement, whether it be just walking, or qi gong, yoga, or tai chi, the brain will respond in a positive way. After all, only we have control over our own brains. We can change those neural pathways. There are plenty of free online videos showing how to practice these healing arts at home.

Brain Zaps

"There's someone in my head, but it's not me."
– Pink Floyd

Just when I thought that I had nothing new to write about, I have discovered that the weird brain sensations I have, which only last for moments, are common among those of us with fibromyalgia. I have had these peculiar short-lived experiences of faintness and brief memory loss followed by dizziness for several years now. It is as though my skull empties for a few seconds; it is somewhat creepy to imagine a skull without a brain!

Many have written that coming off a medication brings about these brain zaps. But I have not come off any medications. Still, I have read that being on Gabapentin can cause them; as mentioned previously, I take only 100 mgs at night. Is this what is causing them? The attacks aren't too frequent but certainly do cause slight dizziness and loss of balance. I have often had electrical shocks throughout my body— this isn't the same thing, nor is it the same as brain fog. I have also had vertigo; it is different from that as well. I wish I had the language to describe the episodes. It's as though my brain loses a second or two into the air and feels disconnected from my body!

It is very frustrating when I lose my sense of balance and veer to the left when I walk. It all seems to be connected to my nervous system so it is reasonable to believe this is common in fibromyalgia. My brain is out of whack. My emotions become dishevelled. Words often fail me and sentence structures are sometimes not intelligible. These little zaps are very peculiar. Fortunately, they aren't frequent and do not last long.

Others have written that changes in temperature can cause brain zaps. This may be true as changes in the environment affect those of us with fibromyalgia. But this isn't the complete answer. The causes seem to be unknown although it is definitely connected to the nervous system. Like fibromyalgia itself, the problem is too many symptoms with too few remedies available. There is little doubt in my mind that these zaps are also part of anxiety episodes. It is the root cause I keep coming back to for answers.

Cognitive and Somatic Sensitization

"If you are experiencing strange symptoms that no one seems
to be able to explain, they could be arising from a traumatic
reaction to a past event that you may not even remember."
– Peter A. Levine

Two words that are now often used in conjunction with fibromyalgia are *cognitive sensitization* and *somatic sensitization*. I have been exploring the research in this direction for the past couple of years and have recently had another "aha" moment. With regards to cognitive sensitization, because of the excessive degree of empathy for others and fear and anxiety for ourselves there is vivid brain activity in the amygdala. People with fibromyalgia worry excessively and our attention to health-related information is extremely high. Our pain and that of others poses increased threats which affect somatic sensitization, that is, increased reactivity of the nervous system. In turn, this sensitization lowers the pain threshold and affects pain tolerance; the consequence is that fibromyalgia syndrome often develops.

How does cognitive sensitization affect us? The answer lies in our pasts, when we may have experienced trauma that the brain won't let us forget, in an attempt to protect us from being hurt again. Its warnings may be acute enough to cause panic attacks and feelings of impending death.

According to Peter Levine, author of *Waking the Tiger,* a study of the effects of past trauma, "The result, sadly, is that many of us become riddled with fear and anxiety and are never fully able to feel at home with ourselves or our world" (21). When our nervous systems are in a state of hyper-arousal, we become overly sensitive to bad news as well as external stimuli like harsh light, loud sounds, and weather conditions. We have difficulty with sleep and processing stressful situations, we startle easily and we are hyper-vigilant. Sometimes our panic is caused by triggers which we might not even recognize.

Social neuroscience has explored the brain activity of many types of people and yet very few studies I could find have been done on the overactive brains of those of us with fibromyalgia. Our tendency to interpret and be in tune with verbal and non-verbal cues of others and be usually in a state of hyper-vigilance is worthy of serious research. As mentioned earlier, many of us with fibromyalgia are in caregiving roles such as nurses. We are addicted to giving care and empathy to others, with the resultant overstimulation. One of the women I interviewed years ago, Valerie, said that she can cry easily and that she is "very emotional and I am hurt easy, like I'm not a fighter. I don't like fights and I don't like arguments." With this high degree of sensitivity, symptoms develop easily. She attributed her fibromyalgia onslaught to stress at work and a car accident which causes symptoms to flare up.

The sudden surge of extreme fearfulness, inability to swallow, heart pounding, shortness of breath, tingling sensations, diarrhea, and feelings of being in danger can develop anywhere and at any time. We are chronic worriers for ourselves and for others, leading to catastrophic thinking. Being afraid of fear itself is what leads to panic attacks. We dwell on things (we are *dwellers*) and we fret (*fretters*). When did these symptoms first begin to take shape in our psyche?

As Levine and Robert Scaer (*The Body Bears the Burden*) have written, we have been subject to psychological trauma that produces bodily sensations that feel like those of a bona fide disease, when what we are actually experiencing is the brain's ongoing response to the initial trauma. We can change those brain pathways if only those who are quick to medicate us or find a cause that is not psycho-social in nature were supportive in our quest to find ways to heal ourselves. Both Levine and Scaer are pioneers in this respect and their work brings hope, rather than resignation, to those of us with this central sensitization. Without hope, what is there? We need to temper the hope that we will be cured with the realization that we are the ones responsible for rebuilding a healthy relationship with our central nervous system, and not expecting anyone else to do it for us. We should remember that cognitive function is shaped over a lifetime and that we can begin today.

Sleep Disturbances

"Trauma is so arresting that traumatized people
will focus on it compulsively."
– Peter Levine

Are sleep disturbances a cause or a symptom of fibromyalgia? I think they are both. Nighttime is when the unconscious mind relives the upsetting events of the day which can be frightening for those of us with a sensitive nature. Our anxiety level is extremely high. The usual advice for getting a good night's sleep often does not work; this includes going to sleep at the same time each night, not taking naps during the day, avoiding caffeine and sugary foods, listening to soft music before going to bed, not watching TV in bed, and being sure the bedroom is not too hot or too cold.

In spite of our best attempts to entice it, sleep is usually elusive for many of us. Monica said, "I have times that either I'm very tired and probably staying awake for days." Another woman I interviewed, Marg, reported that she has "a hard time sleeping, or some nights when I go to sleep, I feel that I've slept all night but when I get up in the morning... I'm tired again, just like I haven't slept."

It is little wonder that sleep disturbances cause many other symptoms, among them *anosognosia* (temporary forgetfulness) which many of us experience as brain fog. The effects of protracted sleep disturbances eventually catch up with us. As Monica noted, "There's times that there's conversations that apparently, I was taking part in... but I have no recollection of the conversation."

There are many kinds of sleep disturbances. Some of us suffer from every one of them. I began having night terrors when I first started Catholic school at age 5, and the nuns told us stories of being responsible for killing

Christ because we were born with original sin on our souls. Of course, this frightened us and made the entire class cry. Today, I recognize the serious trauma this experience was for me and my classmates. We were warned about sin and hell from the first day. I would hyperventilate at night and lose my breath. I was afraid to go to sleep and often fainted. I began sleep walking. It was the time of the polio scare and this added to our fears. World War Two had not yet ended the year I began school, and we were afraid our fathers would be sent away and killed in the war. Indeed, there was much to be anxious about. In addition, my parents were extremely fearful people; before he died in his 90s my father had been diagnosed as with borderline personality disorder, a condition which has added to my lifelong anxiety. The additional traumas of my adult life are too many to document here, but most of us have experienced traumas of one sort or another, many of which can of course affect our sleep.

Going to bed at night has never been a peaceful or relaxing experience for me. I usually awake often and the fibro pain is always present. I have tried many relaxing techniques and meditation before going to bed, and lately I avoid newspapers and the news. The depressing mix of politics, climate change, the economy and health scares heighten our anxieties. Even much of the new music we hear is often grating to our brains. We are warned hourly about everything that could possibly go wrong in our lives and are never taught to relax or look at life joyfully.

All decades have their demons to frighten and alarm us. What is different now is that we are instantly and graphically aware of disasters, thanks to global news coverage. Every news clip warning us about our health ends warnings to the fight or flight part of our brains and causes more hypervigilance. It is little wonder that conditioned as we fibro sufferers are to take on these alarms, the nighttime unconscious brain is even more hyperactive and alarmed. Past or present traumas in our lives incite the nervous system to respond to worry, stimulation and/or excitement.

To prove this point, I glanced recently at a newspaper. I saw headlines about war and Covid, homelessness, poverty and shooting massacres. I could feel the anxiety creeping up on me. Instead of reading more bad news, I picked up a newspaper clipping of a few years ago about Captain Trevor Greene, who suffered a severe brain injury while serving in the Canadian Armed Forces in Afghanistan. He spoke of "retraining [his] brain," to regain old function. "It is neuroplasticity," he explained in an interview. He said he can "almost feel new pathways forming." The article went on to say, "The neuroplastic revolution as some call it, stems from discoveries in the 1960s and 1970s that showed how the brain physically changes as we learn, think and move." Captain Greene spoke about how it takes a lot of willpower to retrain the brain. But his on-going success story is one of courage and discipline. It was inspiring and I know without doubt that those writings about neuroplasticity are intensely relevant to fibromyalgia. We **can** retrain our brains, particularly with regard to sleep patterns.

I wish though that I had easy answers about disturbed sleep patterns. Generally, these are the tips I try to follow, hoping to retrain my brain and form new maps:

1) I try to remember that *occasionally* I may have a good sleep of at least four or five hours and not awaken once.
2) I "de-catastrophize." I have written elsewhere about our tendency to feed into negativity about our pain, lack of sleep and fatigue and to try not to imagine the worst. This only makes our sleep more troublesome. Telling ourselves the sky is not falling is an excellent way to smile at ourselves.
3) I only go to bed when sleepy. Many of us think that if we go to bed earlier, we will have better sleep. That usually isn't true.
4) Try melatonin before bed as it is a natural product and is very helpful for some, although not for me.
5) Try not to nap during the day.
6) Have a snack of something that has tryptophan in it. Eat a banana or try warm milk.
7) Avoid stimulants such as alcohol, which at first may make one sleepy but after it wears off, causes stimulation.
8) Use your bed for only sleeping (or sex), not for reading or watching TV.
9) Don't be a clock watcher (my very worst habit!)
10) Make sure you are not too hot or too cold.

If none of these works, don't be afraid to use a low-dose prescribed sleep medication for a short period of time. Imagine yourself having a restful sleep and follow this positive thought throughout the day. Give your brain a hopeful message! The amygdala, that little part of the brain that affects those of us with fibromyalgia so intensely, needs to receive positive messages to relax and allow us to sleep.

We have to train our brains to believe that we do not have to be on guard during the night. We **can** learn to relax and think of sleep as a safe time to rejuvenate our tired muscles. It takes discipline. We have to remind ourselves that we do occasionally have a good night sleep. Find a comedy show that will bring laughter, listen to soothing music, avoid drama or news on TV, and focus on the bodily sensations that are evoked as we begin to think about the act of sleeping. We can also meditate, breathe deeply and remind ourselves, as my spouse says, "It's time to go off duty."

Fibromyalgia, Chronic Fatigue, and Related Disorders

"Everybody gets so much information all day long
that they lose their common sense."
– Gertrude Stein

To write that I am frustrated, angry, and discouraged over the recent hoopla in the news from the U.S. Institute of Medicine (IOM) report on chronic fatigue syndrome is to be putting it mildly. As is usual with someone who has CFS and fibromyalgia, I awoke several times last night. During those wakeful periods I wanted to write a protest to what I read in the report.

The IOM states that CFS should now be regarded as a **disease**. I write this knowing that the majority of my readers want their condition to be regarded as such so that a medication can be taken and the condition neatly cured. But as I have repeatedly written over many years, this cluster of symptoms which make up a syndrome cannot be "cured" with the usual allopathic (conventional) or alternative medicines. It is far more complex than that. Hunts for viral, bacterial and hormonal causes for CFS and fibromyalgia have been on-going for many decades. I had hoped that we had put these dead ends behind us but wonder now if this trend is going to be re-invented.

The first indication of the awakening of American health experts to the reality of CFS and FMS came to my attention in a *Globe and Mail* article on CFS by André Picard, a writer whom I respect and admire tremendously. While the *f* word (fibromyalgia) is only mentioned once in the article, it is clearly aligned with chronic fatigue. In fact, there may be quadruplets involved here if we combine multiple chemical sensitivities (mentioned by Picard) and PTSD with CFS and FMS. Happily, Picard calls both CFS and FMS disorders, not diseases, something I have long done myself.

My second sighting of this American report was on February 21, 2015 on the CBC news. So now, after decades of the sufferings of millions of people worldwide, the voices of those of us with several of these invisible, but similar disorders will be legitimated. It seems that the IOM has been tasked by the U.S. Department of Health and Human Services, the National Institute of Health, the Agency for Healthcare Research and Quality, the Centers for Disease Control and Prevention, the Food and Drug Administration, the Social Security Administration, all to examine the evidence base for CFS. What on earth are they to do? Are CFS and FMS just *now* being discovered? What do they hope to find that wasn't explored decades ago?

To begin, let's explore the links between CFS and FMS. I have searched, researched and contemplated the relationships between the two as well as what I once called Gulf War Syndrome, shell shock, battle fatigue (now called post traumatic stress disorder) and the elusive multiple chemical sensitivities, all of which are invisible and said to affect women more commonly than men (with the notable exception of PTSD). None of these conditions can be diagnosed with standard medical tests.

What are the commonalities among the four dis-eases of CFS, FMS, MCS and PTSD? The Picard article mentions five main common symptoms:

1) An inability to engage in pre-illness levels of activity that persists for at least six months, accompanied by fatigue. Many symptoms can be traced back to traumatic events such as car accidents, violence, and other situations that cause the nervous system to go into hyper-arousal. Our spirit becomes delicate, we become keenly observant of ourselves and our environment.

2) The worsening of symptoms after any type of exertion (physical, mental or emotional). This post-exercise malaise is seen as key. This symptom is highly evident in both CFS and FMS but can also be seen with MCS and PTSD.

3) Un-refreshing sleep is common to all four disorders.
4) Cognitive impairment (brain fog) Cluttered thinking, inability to remember words, and trouble structuring sentences are common manifestations of these impairments.
5) The inability to stand upright for other than short periods of time, a symptom known as "orthostatic intolerance" which is extremely common in CFS and FMS and may or may not affect the other two disorders.

I have suggested elsewhere in this book that perhaps the "long haulers" or sufferers of "long Covid" have somewhat the same kind of syndrome as FMS and the other disorders. I put forth that idea very, very tentatively as so much is not known about Covid-19 except that it has produced a collective anxiety in the world, resulting in feelings of doom which find us scrolling hour by hour and day by day for new information. However, some of the reported symptoms of long Covid include brain fog, trouble breathing, crushing fatigue, headaches, anxiety and depression, generalized pain, sleep disturbances... sound familiar? Researchers are exploring something they know exists but is invisible; the ends of an obscure spectrum of symptoms, trying to make sense of disparate pieces of information just as they do with fibromyalgia, attempting to build something out of thin air.

These are all "medically unexplained illnesses" with symptoms that are common to all and cannot be separated from one another.

I liken the nervous system of those of us with all these invisible syndromes to an elastic band which has been stretched to its limit. We are never completely cured of this highly sensitive nervous system— it's a work in progress. Whether our condition was caused by nature or nurture cannot be proven. We can only work with the hand we have been dealt. Almost all of the hundreds of people, mostly women, who made comments on my blogs, or who I have interviewed personally have been overly empathetic, intuitive, and caregivers in one form or another. I have not been surprised at the number of nurses who have FMS and CFS, and those from the LGBTQ+ community, racial minorities, as well as other marginalized people whose lives have been filled with trauma. I cannot imagine the pain and suffering from the First Nations families who directly or indirectly encountered the residential schools; these are collective pains. People of colour face racism every day and are in a state of high alert even when walking on the street. Women, the disabled, and the elderly are afraid of going out alone at night and fear for their safety. The list of the vulnerable are endless and we suffer from an abundance of caution.

Some say that after a period of time CFS can be cured without lasting effects. I cannot attest to that, but I can say that those of us with FMS have lifelong challenges, particularly if they are dealing with fragility and other characteristics that make them more physically susceptible to violence. I confess to not hearing from men in the military or in other dangerous professions about their PTSD. I can only speculate that these are highly sensitive men whose nervous systems have been stretched beyond endurance and were in highly volatile life-threatening situations.

Chronic fatigue syndrome has long been considered a disease labelled as myalgic encephalomyelitis (ME); by so labelling this condition as a disease, a person then believes that it is possible to find a cure. For that reason, I generally use the term *chronic fatigue* as it is easier for the general public to understand. The symptoms of CFS and FMS are the same: both are fleeting at times, and there are fairly good days and very bad days. The fatigue that accompanies them is not like tiredness, but rather, crushing fatigue. On very bad days I can hardly get up from the sofa, and to accomplish anything other than going from a comfortable chair to the sofa requires too much energy. It is not like feeling tired at the end of the day. Rather it is like wondering how my body can feel so depleted. Luckily, for me it is episodic while for others it is constant.

One of the women I previously interviewed, Jill, described the extreme fatigue she experienced while trying to keep up with the activities of her day-to-day life: "Every now and then I will go out to maybe a dance, because I love music and I love to dance. But, at the end of the night, I pay for it. By the time I leave there my body has run out of steam. I can hardly walk up the stairs. And of course, the next day, don't look for me, you know because I'm in bed— my body has to recuperate. And you just learn to live with it because you know the next day you just can't function. Your hips ache, your knees ache and sometimes your words don't come out properly, you sound like a babbling idiot. Your concentration is just not there and you just plain feel awful."

I refer the reader to the work of Dr. Ellie Stein from Calgary, Alberta, Canada: http://www.eleanorsteinmd.ca and her pain groups; they have resulted in research into chronic fatigue and fibromyalgia which is very helpful; in particular, I am impressed with her work on neuroplasticity, which offers perhaps the greatest hope for sufferers of both conditions.

Sensitivity and Empathy

"Men are from Earth; women are from Earth. Deal with it."
– George Carlin

A favourite comedian of mine, George Carlin, died few years ago and I miss his humour. While I obviously agree with Carlin's view that both men and women are from Earth, I cannot be quite so cavalier in considering many known differences between the sexes. Sensitivity and empathy, for example, are human emotions that are often expressed very differently by men, women, gays, lesbians, and trans people; this expression affects or may even be responsible for fibromyalgia.

So, the first issue to be explored is the relationship between these close relatives, sensitivity and empathy. Basically, sensitivity means being receptive to the verbal and non-verbal cues of others as well as sensory sensitivity. Empathy is the ability to identify with another person's feelings. People who are said to be *in*sensitive to others are thought to lack empathy, whereas those who are *non*empathetic are said to lack sensitivity. However, these descriptors are still not so clear cut. In a negative sense people can be sensitive in a highly intuitive way but lack in appropriate empathetic behaviours, such as those who abuse others while being aware of /sensitive to the pain they are causing.

Within the past few decades, the term "emotional intelligence" has been used to both critique IQ tests and to expand the definition of human intelligence beyond mere academic ability. In this view, a person may have a high IQ, but without emotional intelligence, high IQ is less noteworthy. People who have a high degree of emotional intelligence are said to have empathy for the feelings of others and insight regarding how others think; in short, they are highly sensitive. They can easily understand group dynamics and the individual feelings of others. The term *emotional intelligence* has been used in both corporate and academic settings with differing perspectives about whether or not it is useful as an endeavour to understand human capacity and emotions. My intent is not to discuss this in any greater detail but to show that sensitivity and empathy are now thought to be key to how people relate to one another.

As mentioned previously, it is my belief that persons with fibromyalgia, and women in particular, have a highly over-developed sensitivity therefore experience *too much* empathy for others. These emotions become a liability in that the inability to shut down our feelings for others to a degree that is safe for us, prevents us from the recognition and understanding of the effect this inability has on our own bodies and nervous systems. Sometimes called "empaths," we are people who take on other people's emotions as though they were our own. We are not able to relax into the state that is necessary to maintain a healthy body because we accumulate emotions of our own and those of others. In addition, we are people who are often high-achieving, highly motivated, and high-energy.

When the nervous system becomes continually aroused, perhaps due to taking on the experiences of others or because of an accident, illness or injury of our own, we may develop chronic fibromyalgia.

Here are some questions you can ask if you recognize yourself in this description of the highly-sensitive, empathetic person: when you see someone in pain, do you almost experience it yourself? If someone stumbles, do you have a wrenching feeling in your stomach as if you too were about to fall (while others may get a chuckle out of the scenario)? Do movies with loud noises and great stimulation evoke agitation in you rather than enjoyment? If you answered "yes" to these questions, you may have a predisposition to an overactive nervous system that is a hallmark of FMS.

Why does it seem as though women are more prone to developing fibromyalgia than men? Or at least why do more women report their concerns to physicians and receive the diagnosis of FMS than men? It seems likely that it may be due to the differences between the genders (of which there is acknowledged gender fluidity and several genders) and the ways in which sensitivity and empathy are experienced and expressed. However, we often focus on the differences between men and women rather than observing similarities. Not all women are sensitive and empathetic nor are all men insensitive and lacking in empathy. Expectations that all women should be nurturing and caring while men should be tough and non-intuitive is limiting. The jury is still out trying to assess how many men suffer from fibromyalgia. Furthermore, do trans persons have a change in their sensitivity and empathy dispositions?

All this brings me to this point: sensitivity must be accompanied by empathy to be considered a positive trait. Furthermore, I believe that those with both, but too much of either, over-stimulate their nervous systems, ignore their own needs, and often develop fibromyalgia. Human emotions are complex and culturally defined. More questions keep arising for me as shades of gray appear instead of black and white answers.

Anton St. Marten writes that to feel intensely is "the trademark of the truly alive and compassionate." We have been conditioned to believe that the person who is highly empathetic and sensitive is weak; in fact, it may be more accurate to say that our society is dysfunctional and often lacking in empathy.

People with fibromyalgia additionally suffer from being misunderstood. A January 22, 2018 article published online in Fibromyalgia News Today and titled "Personality Disorders Prevalent Among Fibromyalgia Patients, Study Suggests" shows how those with FMS are labelled by the medical establishment. The article's author, Alice Melão, reviews the medical literature on the condition and reports on their findings that those with fibromyalgia are "exhausting to manage," "perfectionists," and "demanding." Furthermore, "Personality disorders such as obsessive-compulsive, avoidance and histrionic behaviors, are prevalent comorbidities among patients with diagnosed fibromyalgia." I was aghast when I read this article and felt empathy for readers who were hurt by this depiction of their personality. As one commentator wrote, "These articles are not only useless, they are damaging."

From this review, it would appear that people with fibromyalgia are hysterical, difficult to manage, and obsessive-compulsive. This is certainly not the profile I would give to the thousands of readers of my blogs, who definitely had something in common with one another, though not a personality disorder. Our commonality is hyper-empathetic sensitivity in a world gone awry.

Celebrities like Lady Gaga and Morgan Freeman have spoken publicly about their struggles with FMS, and it is to be hoped that their disclosures will help remove some of the stigma surrounding the dis-ease. No doubt there are many more public figures who have not disclosed that they too have the same symptoms.

I do not see myself as a "high-maintenance" person, as some of the medical literature might suggest. As a child, and later as a responsible mother, wife and professor, I was never considered "difficult to manage." I was generally compliant, easy to get along with, and certainly an obedient child. More to the point, I have never been in the least bit obsessive-compulsive nor hysterical. Additionally, I have never been considered a perfectionist; in fact, (and unfortunately for my spouse) the exact opposite again. So why is it that those of us with FMS are considered people with similar "personality disorders," a damning label? Is it because we have an invisible disorder and therefore our health challenges are considered suspect? Is it because the majority of us reporting to health professionals are women and highly sensitive? Why is it that the military who have PTSD (a version of fibromyalgia) have a different name for the same symptoms? We all have great compassion for the veterans who suffer from that syndrome and do not denigrate them.

The question now is to ask researchers if we have a disorder or rather, an intense desire to help others to the detriment of ourselves? Consider this: why do so many nurses and social workers have fibromyalgia? Why are so many military personnel suffering from PTSD? We see, hear and anticipate the pain of others in these overly empathetic minds of ours to the extent that anxiety becomes second nature, particularly as we had not developed a hard shell in our earlier years. We are highly intuitive, much more than the general public. Is this a disorder or a gift? Why does fibromyalgia continue to have a psychiatric label that is considered to be shameful?

FMS and Mental Health

"My friend…care for your psyche…know thyself, for once we
know ourselves, we may learn how to care for ourselves."
– Socrates

As we have seen, fibromyalgia is not easily diagnosed by standard scientific tests. Many physicians press the 18 so-called "trigger points" on the body and if 11 or more are tender, a loose diagnosis is made. However, as discussed previously, the pain of FMS waxes and wanes, which makes us question the accuracy of a diagnosis. If a broad spectrum of symptoms is present, including pain, chronic fatigue, sleeplessness, depression, and chronic anxiety, accompanied by tender points, then a more definite label of fibromyalgia is made. But only if these symptoms persist for more than six months.

The official diagnostic wording made in 1990 by a committee of the American College of Rheumatologists, led by Dr. Fredrick Wolfe, suggested that fibromyalgia is not an actual disease, but is a response to stress, depression and anxiety.

As mentioned previously, those who suffer from FMS have often been treated as mentally ill people who cannot manage their lives. One could say that FMS is as much an emotional dis-ease as a physical one. Those with FMS often resort to mood-altering medications in their quest to feel better.

Nonetheless, antidepressants and anti- anxiety medications **can** help those who are challenged with daily symptoms and need a stop-gap measure while using other therapeutic strategies to overcome their struggles.

The book *Diagnosis, Therapy and Evidence Conundrums in Modern American Medicine*, by Gerald N Grot and Allan V Horwitz points out the lack of pathobiology in FMS and CFS. The pharmaceutical industry has been the victor in all of this and we have fed into it unwillingly in our effort to alleviate our suffering and obtain some degree of relief. So many people write to me citing the numerous medications they are taking. The side effects are frightening.

The question of whether being a highly sensitive person is a mental health issue or not is complex, but to stigmatize ourselves is worse than admitting we suffer from anxiety and/or depression. No matter how strongly our nervous system reacts to stress, we have nothing to be ashamed of. This is especially true in these Covid times when many of us are suffering from anxiety, alienation, social isolation, and loss. We live in chaotic times and feel these emotions very deeply.

The intriguing research and theoretical debates about the brain are related to the mystery of how we develop consciousness, and in the case of fibromyalgia, how does our consciousness relate to our real-life experiences of pain? Philosophers, neuroscientists, psycho-neurologists, sociologists, and neuro-ethicists are studying this mind/body relationship and the nature of consciousness. For those who are interested in finding out how our consciousness manages to communicate to our brain that we are in pain, the book *The Quest for Consciousness* by Christof Koch may provide some answers in language that is easy to understand.

I read recently that with the work of the scientists who are making tremendous advances in understanding the brain that we will soon be able to look into our own brains and engage in individualized brain therapy. Imagine! We will be able to scan for both positive and negative psycho-social emotions, just as we tried to read our own minds in earlier times with the mood rings of the 1950s and biofeedback in the 1980s. While this scanning of our brains may seem frightening to many, including neuro-ethicists, it could be a relief to many, especially those who frequently experience thoughts of disaster from their hyperactive amygdalae. Maybe the time will come when we can change those impulses that lead to negative thoughts and images through mechanical means. In the meantime, rather than hoping for others to work with our thoughts and emotions, we can learn to become our own change agents by making lifestyle choices to calm our own nervous systems down.

The Pain is in the Brain: Are Mind and Brain the Same?

"Memory, the warder of the brain."
– William Shakespeare

My learning about the brain began with my physiotherapist, who brought me to a path which I had never travelled down before, that is, to explore the relationship of pain and the brain, rather than looking simply at fibromyalgia as the result of a hyper-aroused nervous system. Let's begin with a brief discussion about how the nervous system and the brain work.

There are approximately 100 billion nerve cells in the brain which is amazing considering that it weighs only about 3 pounds. lbs. The brain is a large network of interconnected neurons and the communication that takes place between them. A synapse is the connection between two neurons. Important information is filtered through the synapses to consciousness, and it may amplify the signal to hyper-awareness, leading to the heightened awareness of pain that afflicts those of us with fibromyalgia. In short, the neurons become scrambled!

The spinal cord and the brain make up the central nervous system. The brain takes messages to the peripheral nervous system which controls the limbs and organs of the body. Within this system is the autonomic nervous system which affects the sympathetic and parasympathetic nervous systems. The sympathetic system controls the "fight or flight" warning which secretes extra adrenaline and cortisol into the bloodstream. In those of us with fibromyalgia, the brain keeps repeatedly warning this system to be fearful. Our nervous systems become hyper-aroused and *freezing* occurs, which is another aspect to the fight or flight concept. The brain does not allow the parasympathetic system to do its proper job of "rest and relaxation." But we can retrain our brain to overcome this chronic hyper-arousal! That is the wonderful news that is exciting to neuroscientists and psycho-neurologists who have a few decades ago uncovered the *plasticity* of the brain. New emotions can be learned in a process which is not any different from learning a skill like playing chess or tennis. It requires time and discipline but with practice the brain is built to allow us to train for positive emotions, rather than the painful ones that plague sufferers of fibromyalgia.

Here is a conundrum: what, in fact, is the difference between the brain and the mind? Are they the same thing? The physiotherapist says that "the mind emerges as the function of the physical structures of the brain." It might even be plausible to suggest that there isn't even a mind, since it cannot be seen and all that there may be is a brain! Some believe that the mind is our experiences and the ability to become aware of such things as our surroundings. It is our consciousness and our thoughts. Within this view, the mind comes after the brain. It embraces the higher functions of the brain such as our personality, reason, memory, and emotions.

So, is it possible for us to find ways to circumvent the mind and focus on the brain itself before it gives those messages of pain to our conscious mind? Can we give the mind different messages? Or even more daringly, is it plausible that the mind is non-existent and maybe we should be concentrating only on the brain, which in fact does those functions that are said to be in the mind?

The brain itself is biological matter and can be found and touched. The mind cannot be seen by anyone, nor is it biological. It reminds me that when we hear about the body-mind connection or body-mind-spirit, what we are actually talking about is more concrete. Neither the mind nor the spirit (or soul) can be seen or touched. I prefer instead to think about the connection between the body, the brain, and the emotions; in this triad, only emotions cannot be seen or touched, but they can actually be measured to some degree. The body and the brain are tangible. It is those biological aspects of pain which we hope to change so that the brain receives different messages than it has had before, ones that bring about more hopeful and happier emotions. I recognize that there may be criticisms about letting go of the concept of a *mind* and instead focussing only on the brain. This will be so particularly in the Buddhist tradition which suggests that there is a distinct difference between the brain and the mind. Nonetheless, I believe there is a more concrete aspect to embrace in this search for the impact of pain on the mind.

The brain has a lifelong ability to reorganize neural pathways and has the ability to change with learning (via *brain plasticity*). The advances in research that have been conducted have revealed that the brain can change in response to experiences. It can be trained by learning new ways of *responding* rather than the constant *reacting* to stimuli (particularly to the real or perceived needs of others) which is common in fibromyalgia. It isn't easy but with awareness it can be done! In short, the brain is not static; it can be retrained. Thanks to increased awareness of our brain's ability to change, we have learned that we can change the pattern of our overly empathetic emotions which appear to be solidified within us (for those with fibromyalgia). We can learn to differentiate between appropriately compassionate and empathetic responses, and overly empathetic reactions to others which tax our nervous systems.

The anxiety and stressful emotions which plague our every day lives are in our brains but can be retrained to send different messages to become happy and peaceful, while minimizing the over-stimulation of the adrenals, thereby reducing pain in the brain. Rather than repeating these same patterns of responses to pain brought about by stored memories, new neural pathways can bring about needed changes to our thoughts and emotions. It is the brilliant writing of Diane Jacobs which has recently brought me to these insights. Here are some of her recommended steps towards self-regulating our condition:

1) Reconceptualize the problem.
2) Help the nervous system to calm itself down.
3) Employ psychological techniques. One of her important pieces of advice is to remember that hurt does not equal harm and this is important for those of us who have persistent pain which changes in location and nature. Jacobs writes that "Letting pain be our guide actually increases our risk of developing ongoing pain-related anxiety and avoidance."

One of the women I interviewed for my first book, Katy, described the experience of taking control of her health rather than allowing her fibromyalgia to control her life: "I was diagnosed in one shot with a family physician who knew a lot about the condition and said from day one almost 'You are going to have to find your own way with this condition.' I was actively encouraged to find my way."

How to build new neural pathways? The Buddhist Kalu Rinpoche has suggested, "Take a simple activity that requires attention but not much intellectual effort and do it again and again." (That, by the way, is why I took up a new project of hand-sewing a quilt, something I have never done before).

Neuroplasticity, brain mapping, the interconnectedness of various parts of the brain with the body, a more in-depth understanding of the difference between the mind and the brain, and more comprehensive knowledge about brain science are a bit beyond me at this point. But I am certain that with a deeper scientific knowledge of the brain and its ability to change, we are on the right path to a greater understating of many illnesses and dis-eases. The future is with more evidence-based knowledge of the complexity of the brain.

Gender and Fibromyalgia

"The happiest women, like the happiest nations, have no history."
– George Eliot

I have based my theory about why more women than men are diagnosed with fibromyalgia upon a feminist analysis of the political and cultural roles of women in societies in general, both historically and at present. However, now that more people are learning that gender is socially constructed and is much less binary than originally thought, the issue of gender has become a complex one and not as straightforward as it was when I wrote my first book. I would like to acknowledge the change that has taken place in society and in my thinking in the years since that book was published.

What in fact is a woman? Does the term apply only to those born with female sexual organs? For many, the term "woman" now includes transgendered people.

These days, I look less often at statistics regarding the ratio of women to men with FMS because I believe that fibromyalgia is a catch-all term that includes all genders who suffer from chronic pain and fatigue. It is also a condition that is under-reported by those of all genders. Millions of people, young and old, of different races, levels of privilege and genders suffer from fibromyalgia worldwide.

The concept of fibromyalgia developed as more and more women began to speak out about similar characteristics and symptoms which caused physicians to believe that it was a condition that afflicted more women than men. There isn't any way to accurately determine how much of the population of any country has fibromyalgia. In many countries, there isn't even a term for the condition, and many self-identified men have been hesitant to report their symptoms to a health care professional for fear of being seen as less masculine.

It is well known that those who identify as women are more likely to seek medical attention for both their families and themselves than are men.[7] Furthermore, women who are born with female physical attributes are generally more sensitive to bodily changes and other nuances that are often difficult to describe. An example of this is the reported sense of impending doom that women often experience in the weeks or days before a heart attack (unfortunately, I can attest to that). Yet, when women mention to their health care providers symptoms that should be directly attributed to heart disease, there is still a general misconception that heart disease is primarily a man's condition. Conversely, when a woman discusses her chronic pain, fatigue and other symptoms with her physician, the label of fibromyalgia is more readily applied. If a man admits to having chronic pain, the affected areas are more likely to be vigorously examined and attributed to, for example, a disk, muscular strain, and so on.

Why is it that women and men are treated so differently within the health care systems, in particular with regard to chronic pain, fatigue, anxiety, and depression? It is true that fibromyalgia is not life-threatening, but given the large numbers of people affected by the condition, why is it still believed that FMS is primarily a woman's condition? Even more to the point, why is it that researchers are keen to explore what they perceive as problems within the woman's body which *causes* fibromyalgia?

I have written extensively about the highly sensitive person and fibromyalgia, which I believe to be the same as the highly anxious person. This in turn, is seen as an issue of mental instability that is associated with women as more women report symptoms of emotional distress and take more mood-altering medications than men.

Globally and historically, women have suffered more frequently from sexism, domestic abuse, crime, ageism, racism, rape, sexual abuse, incest, poverty, and economic inequality. It is little wonder that women suffer more from lifelong anxiety and their spirits are often broken. The question I often ask myself is why anxiety and fibromyalgia have become

---

[7] I use the terms "men" and "women" in the traditional sense—that is, referring to those born with male or female physical characteristics.

medicalized and are thought to be shameful when they are the direct result of women's socially-constructed roles in life.

Do the pressures of beauty and fashion, sexual activity, social structures that are constraining, and the "glass ceiling" effect in the workplace perpetuate women's lifelong struggles with anxiety, even in the most "stable" and privileged environments? Even more to the point, what groups are left out in discussions about fibromyalgia: people of colour, LGBTQ+ communities, those living in war-torn countries, homeless people, and other disadvantaged groups who suffer from this syndrome? Surely their pain and fatigue are even more underreported than that of more privileged groups, such as white men.

Some physical therapists (physiotherapists) believe that fibromyalgia pain is caused by hypermobility of joints. While their view is somewhat interesting, it has not been my experience with the women I have interviewed who suffer from FMS. Other than among certain PTs, I have not heard others suggest that this could be a cause of this painful syndrome. It does appear though that it is an end result that joints become less mobile as mobility is decreased: "rest means rust." Are women noted for having hypermobility of joints?

Some endocrinologists believe there is a decreased nocturnal level of prolactin (a single-chain protein hormone closely related to growth hormone) in women with FMS. Still others believe there is a genetic component in FMS and that some people are more predisposed to developing it. Some are convinced that FMS is due to inadequate thyroid regulation.

Less fruitful for research purposes is the theory that there is a chemical imbalance in the muscles of women with FMS, the pain of which can be explained by a malic acid and magnesium deficiency. While it may be so that there is a chemical imbalance in the muscles of persons with FMS, the question to be asked once more is why this is reported primarily in women.

Chronic fatigue among women seems to be a focus of interest of late by, among others, the US-based Centers for Disease Control and Prevention. Their primary thrust is that of genetic mutations. And so, the search for medical causes of FMS and CFS continues.

Furthermore, if fibromyalgia is the same as PTSD, don't both affect men and women, trans, and other gender identities as well? Just as there is race-mixing, there is also gender-mixing. None of these issues are clear cut.

As research into the causes of FMS continues, few (if any) suggest that FMS and CFS may occur more frequently in women as a result of oppressive social structures in society which condition women (and some men) to put the needs of others before their own. This sense of always being on duty could result in an over-aroused nervous system. Women of colour, lesbians, bisexual and trans women often live in constant fear of acts of homophobia, racism and transphobia, keeping their nervous systems in a hyper-aroused state.

In addition to the highly sensitive temperamental profile of many FMS sufferers, we can add the additional characteristic of being high-energy and high-achieving. In my first book, I interviewed a woman named Lena who said, "My personality is to push, push, push, push. If I do an amount of work in a certain time, I think, 'oh well, I should have done more.' I know another girl who has fibro and her personality is very, very outgoing and she was pushing herself doing all these volunteer things— 10,000 places at once and she felt bad because she had to stop". It seemed as though the women felt compelled to work until they collapsed with a fibromyalgia flare-up.

The question arises about why fibromyalgia is more prevalent in highly sensitive women and men. The debate about the effects of nature versus nurture on the development of FMS has not yielded specific answers and for awhile I have thought of it as a moot point. As a nurse and sociologist, I have leaned toward the impact of the social environment in early childhood. But as some of the science in human sexuality suggests, there is a relationship between levels of testosterone in utero and the extent to which specific traits are manifested after birth.

Does fibromyalgia occur as a result of an anxious mother who could not easily handle stress and anxiety because she was not herself exposed to enough testosterone, thereby depleting the fetus of sufficient testosterone? Had this fetus had such exposure, would she then be more qualified for the more mechanically-oriented occupations like science and math, as has been suggested?

A Google controversy has brought forth arguments from both sides regarding sexism versus science. The neuroscientist Debra Soh, writing in the *Globe and Mail*,[8] states: "Contrary to what detractors would have you believe, women are on average, higher on neuroticism and agreeableness, and lower in stress tolerance [than men]."

Given the state of the world, it seems likely that women and highly sensitive men are indeed more anxious and less able to effectively handle the chaos and instability which men with high levels of testosterone have created. One need only to watch the news to notice the continued presence of men raising havoc in the world. What have testosterone levels done to those of us with low levels of the hormone? Are we, in general, neurotic, anxious and passively agreeable as Soh suggests? Has that resulted in syndromes of medically unexplained syndromes (MUS) such as fibromyalgia, chronic fatigue syndrome, and PTSD to name a few? Did we develop these syndromes because we have less testosterone or is it because we cannot tolerate the ways in which we women, people of colour, the LGBTQ2+, poor and other disadvantaged groups are being treated? How do we answer all these questions given the hormone taking of transgendered persons?

As with so much about fibromyalgia, we are left with more questions than answers.

---

[8] August 9, 2017, A11

Gay Men and FMS

"I know that you cannot live on hope alone, but
without it, life is not worth living."
– Harvey Milk

Many research studies, from Sweden to the UK and the US, suggest that gay men's brains are symmetrical to those of straight women. In particular, a Swedish study published in the *National Academy of Sciences Journal* supports this finding, although whether or not it is genetic, occurs in the womb, is the result of sex hormones or environmental factors, remains controversial. What hasn't been adequately reported are issues related to brain studies of bisexual or trans-sexual people, so most of these findings are not as clear cut as they originally seemed.

The studies to date regarding women and gay men have mainly focused on the similarities in the area of the brain responsible for storing emotions such as anxiety, in the amygdala, an almond-shaped structure found in each brain hemisphere. The amygdala directs the rest of the brain in response to emotional stimuli, instigating the "fight or flight" response. It is the part of the brain involved in "emotional learning."

As these findings have gained more acceptance in the scientific community —that is, that gay men and straight women have similar responses to emotions like anxiety and also a high degree of empathy—it seems plausible to suggest that fibromyalgia may affect gay men as much as it does women. Since I believe that fibromyalgia is the result of an overstimulated nervous system brought about by social (and subsequently physical) conditions of hypersensitive persons, then it would follow that marginalized groups like gay men, living in an often-homophobic society, would also be greatly susceptible to this condition. Obviously, I am just speculating, in particular since I have not heard from many gay men with fibromyalgia.

There is so much to be yet learned about gender identities; the science has barely begun. But there is hope as more LGBTQ+ communities are demanding answers and equal rights.

I have heard from a young gay man with fibromyalgia who relates his difficult life situation. Both his parents and those of his partner do not accept their relationship and are homophobic. After a car accident he developed fibromyalgia and his subsequent searches for help are numerous. Many of us have been on a similar path: family physician, massage therapist, specialists of every kind… his list seems endless to him. Is he, like many of us, searching for a cure when in fact, the cause is primarily societal and political in nature and of course, biological, since pain is in the brain? These are the issues that distress me as I read sad fibromyalgia tales, though I refuse to give up hope for answers.

The Orchid Child

"The orchid child is the child who shows great sensitivity
and susceptibility to both bad and good environments
in which he or she finds herself or himself."
– Dr. Thomas Boyce

Do you know someone who seems to be an antenna for other people's emotions? Someone who is so finely-attuned to feeling that looking at a painting or listening to a piece of music may bring them easily to tears?

A January 1, 2011 *Globe and Mail* article written by Anne McIlroy entitled "How to raise an 'orchid child' to blossom" has given me a name for this kind of sensitivity. I love the term "orchid child" as it likens the sensitive child to a beautiful hothouse plant. Often used as a symbol for spring and associated with the beauty of women, an orchid is a lovely image to embrace. It has been written that an orchid is a "flower of noble character". An orchid is also a fragile plant that needs just the exact amount of light and nourishment in order to blossom, but not wilt. Orchid children may be labelled with the less poetic "sensory-processing sensitivity."

I read this article with great interest, recognizing my childhood self in the description of the orchid child. Here are some of the ways in which this trait manifests in children, and I invite readers to see if any of these criteria resonate with their own past experiences, too: Did you/do you: "Notice the slightest unusual odour? Prefer quiet play? Complain about scratching clothing, tags in clothes or seams in socks? Startle easily? Perform best when strangers aren't around? Feel things deeply? Notice when others are in distress? Have trouble falling asleep after an exciting day?"

In addition, are you sensitive to pain? A perfectionist? Overly emphatic and emotive? Bothered by noisy places? Without doubt these are the ways in which most people with fibromyalgia would describe themselves. Were those of us with fibromyalgia orchid children?

One of the women I interviewed, Bonnie, spoke of herself in terms reminiscent of an orchid child: "When I had the diagnosis my mother called me a hothouse plant. I've always been labelled as being too sensitive, hyper-sensitive. Too much stimuli bothers me, gets me upset."

While much of the research on orchid children seems to be focused around the genetic code and also on the role of poverty and other environmental vulnerabilities, nothing has been written about these personality characteristics and fibromyalgia. I have a hunch that will soon change as the prevalence of fibromyalgia accelerates in these difficult social, health and economic times and there are more demands for answers to this perplexing condition affecting our sensitive receptors.

On parenting and being parented

"If you look deeply into the palm of your hand, you will
see your parents and all generations of your ancestors. All
of them are alive in this moment. Each is present in your
body. You are the continuation of each of these people."
– Thich Nhat Hanh

It may be impossible to know how much early childhood experiences
are responsible for the development of fibromyalgia in later life. The
issue of parenting styles is a thorny one, and while parent-blaming has
become a common practice in our times, I don't think doing so is helpful.
Who among us had perfect parents? Who among us are perfect parents
ourselves? We are all doing our best! We often do not know all the stories
of our parents and if we have children, they do not know all of ours.

What did our parents know about parenting? Like most of us, they
passed on the values and beliefs they had acquired from their own parents.
Those of my parents' generation believed in a patriarchal, strict household
without much awareness of the psycho-social needs of their children.
Life was difficult for people raised in the Depression era, and many had
struggles that caused overwhelming challenges when they became parents.
School and church were strict and frightening places for their offspring,
as they were for them, and we 1950s kids received little sympathy as we
accepted the status quo without question, as they did.

I still remember the horrors of Catholic school, fainting spells,
hyperventilating at night, sleep walking and nightmares. There was very
little to soothe my nervous system as my mother was herself a fearful
woman and for many years, I was an only child subject to her worries and
anxieties, in effect becoming her mother.

School and church were places which were harmful to my psyche. There I was constantly on guard as a nun in a rage was not to be reckoned with at any cost. I would never have dreamed of rebelling; instead, I became super-vigilant. My parents would not have understood why I began having fainting spells, nor would have many people of that era. I can't blame them. The information we have nowadays can help us understand better what a healthy environment should be like for a child to grow up strong and confident, without living in a state of hypervigilance.

As I raised my own children, I did not know what I know now watching my young grandchildren. I made my own kind of mistakes, as we all do. Like those of us with fibromyalgia, I carried the weight of the world on my shoulders; I felt an intense, even unrealistic degree of obligation to my family of origin as well as to my own children. As a woman, I was viewed as the nurturer, the selfless giver, the compassionate mother. I was always second guessing someone else's needs and would reproach myself for the smallest act of negligence toward what I considered my duty. The cost of such high expectations of self? An over aroused nervous system which was never in a state of rest.

Childhood Conditioning

"Fear-controlled by anxious, fearful parents, these children
often become anxious and fearful themselves." -
— Susan Forward

It seems clear that fibromyalgia and chronic fatigue are caused by early traumatic experiences which only talk therapy will begin to help us unravel. In my own case, I am certain that my childhood experiences have set me up for a lifetime of high anxiety which led to FMS.

It isn't an easy thing for me to do, being "out there" about my struggles. I do not see myself as a victim, and life could have been much more difficult, as it is for many. That my parents loved me, I have no doubt. Their life circumstances were not easy either, and this is not about parent-blaming.

As mentioned earlier, my mother was exceptionally anxious and my father was absent most of the time; he was an angry man, prone to violent outbursts, who felt forced into marriage. My Mum spent every day drinking coffee, smoking, and listening to the radio. My family lived in Montreal, but she could not speak French and did not have any friends or relatives in the city. Because we were English-speaking, we did not fit into our predominantly French neighborhood. It was just my mother and me alone every day without any family or other adults with whom to interact. My mother guarded me closely and lived for my company. I was the one who would buy needed groceries as I learned to speak French at an early age.

I found one girlfriend, Lise, who was French and who became my constant play- mate. I learned to speak French at age three so that we could communicate, though my mother could not communicate with Lise's mother. Being Anglophones meant we were frequently discriminated against, so I did everything in my power not to be noticed as different. I would change my name to a French one if someone in the neighborhood asked me for it. English-speaking people were called "tête carrée," that is, "square head" as a French-language slur against Anglophones in Quebec. I was terrified that I might be found out and called that name, so I always tried to "pass." Lise helped me in my lonely life. As playmates, we were inseparable.

I was forced to go to an English Catholic school at age five and was separated from my only friend who attended a French Catholic school nearby. I had a long trek to school, by streetcar or bus, or on fine days, I walked. I would spend the whole day without Lise, our roller skates and balls, our paper dolls, real dolls, and skipping ropes.

My first day of school will always be remembered for the terror I felt seeing nuns for the first time in my sheltered five-year-old life. Up until this time I had not been in a church as my parents did not attend. I was a quiet, obedient child.

It was an all-girls school, as was common in that era, and I wore a uniform with long stockings that were mandatory. We were all crying. My mother left me as did all the other parents. As soon as the door closed, we were forced to go down on our knees to learn prayers. We were told that the dead man on the huge crucifix was killed because of us and the "original sin" we had been born with. We all sobbed, some of us uncontrollably. Each day before classes we knelt to pray, and before and after recess, and again before lunch break. The same process was enacted after lunch. Catechism was preached and memorized and we had to kiss the feet of the crucifix with Sister swiping the feet after each kiss with what I presume was alcohol, because it was the polio era. The story of the crucifixion haunted me day and night.

The nuns terrified us all. They would walk around with wooden clappers; avoiding having a finger or ear lobe clasped in a clapper was a strong deterrent to misbehaving. But it was the wrath of God we feared the most and the stories of his death. "Holy cards" were handed out to the deserving children. Preparing for my first communion meant I had to begin my weekly confession. Finding sins to confess was a difficult task for a small child. I learned to say by rote:

"I have sinned exceedingly in thought, word, and deed, through my fault, through my fault, through my most grievous fault."

On each *fault* I would rap my chest. I had no idea what my sins were, but I must have had some. I was almost seven by then, living in an almost completely enclosed tiny bed-sitting apartment on a busy street, with a lonely, anxious, terrified mother and only Lise for comfort. What sins had I committed? My mother frequently told me I must never lie to her or God would hear me. I was terrified of him and very obedient. I had no opportunity or inclination to steal. I didn't know any swear words. I didn't understand most of the Ten Commandments. I must have been sin-free, but that was not possible in the Catholic worldview.

In addition to the terrors at school, we all lived with an intense fear of dying of polio, which was still active in the 1940s; one of my classmates had died from it. We were also living in the aftermath of World War Two. There was little joy in life and no grandparents, aunts, uncles, cousins or adult friends to ease the burden.

I began hyperventilating, particularly at bedtime, and my father, when he was at home one night, taught me to breathe in a paper bag during a panic attack which helped calm me somewhat. I was convinced I would die and go to hell.

Furthermore, I began to faint often, particularly before going to school in the morning. Anxiety, panic, hyperventilating and fainting, and living with an anxious parent are all precursors to fibromyalgia. My blue-collar parents would not have known that I needed emotional help, but during those times therapy was not common.

By now I was exceptionally hypersensitive, living with Catholic guilt. It would take a few more years before full-blown fibromyalgia would develop, but the groundwork was laid. Anxiety would become my lifelong companion; nighttime would always be feared; guilt would plague me forever; depression would surface easily; sleep disturbances would haunt me. If only I had been able to talk with a responsible adult! It was an era when there was little understanding of the intensity of a child's fear.

For those of us who have experienced difficult childhoods and can afford to spend time with a therapist, run, don't walk, find someone you can trust. It is at least a beginning step towards an understanding of how fibromyalgia and its associated anxiety and depression along with the physical manifestations first began.

My grown-up years were marked by trauma, poverty, divorce, and being stalked, but many of the details of these stories are too personal to share.

Now in my old age, I have had the great fortune to be married to my soul mate for the past four decades. This has been a factor in my healing from early traumatic experiences.

The "Science" of Fibromyalgia

"Nothing in life is to be feared. It is only to be understood."
– Marie Curie

A few years ago I heard a presentation from a distinguished scientist speaking about fibromyalgia. The audience seemed to be mostly comprised of people with FMS. He referred to fibromyalgia as a "terrible disease." My immediate reaction was negative as I don't believe that fibromyalgia is a disease, but rather a syndrome; he also referred to pain as a disease, which further surprised me. Language is so important to our understanding of this condition; if we feed into this idea of a disease, more and more researchers will continue to search for an elusive and non-existent virus or bacteria or continue the search for hormonal issues, without an emphasis on psycho-social causation.

The presentation focused on how pain changes the physical structure of the brain, but the speaker said nothing about the (to me) far more interesting issue of whether structural changes could be caused by socio-psychological triggers. I would prefer that the focus be on what caused these changes rather than to assume that people with fibromyalgia are born with genetic defects. However, the question about whether or not we are born with unusual brain wiring or we acquire it from our early socialization is one which may never be answered.

There were many aspects of the presentation which I did like; for example, the presenter spoke of pain as that which cannot be measured or objectified and that it is a subjective experience. I have written about this elsewhere and concur with him. The speaker spoke of fibromyalgia as a central nervous system disease, and although I know this to be true, I would have substituted the term "dis-ease." Much of the presentation was too technical for me—and I presume, the audience—to understand fully. What did pique my interest was the discussion about potential causes. Many possibilities were presented: genetic, environmental (among them psychiatric, stress-related, and caused by injury), genetic changes related to neuroticism and the tendency to have negative personality traits, but strangely, none that were sociological. In fact, the entire presentation lacked any psycho-sociological analysis.

The gender issue was not presented except to say that more women than men have fibromyalgia; after a question from the audience, the reply was that women's nervous systems are different from those of men. This of course negates the issue of trans, gay, queer, and non-binary people and fibromyalgia, which I believe is greatly underreported.

So, what conclusions did I draw from that presentation about where FMS science is leading us? Certainly, drugs are being tested and fibromyalgia is being investigated scientifically within the realm of pain research. The drug research focuses on alleviating pain while minimizing side effects on the brain.

The acceptance of FMS by the scientific community as an expression of heightened central nervous system sensitivity is a positive development. What requires more research is the sociological dimension of FMS and its connection to the hypersensitive person. Further, we need to expand our vision of FMS as a condition affecting all genders, not only women, whose bodies have been historically medicalized. We need to understand why fibromyalgia is underreported in men. We cannot continue to view fibromyalgia as a disease.

I'm willing to bet that there is a huge cadre of those of us with fibromyalgia who would be willing to take part in brain research. We want to change our brains and calm our nervous systems! However, given that fibromyalgia is seen by many as a disease entity, our bodies will continue to be medicalized and psycho-social conditions that precipitate fibromyalgia will be ignored. After all, there isn't as much grant money given to scientists for research into the societal conditions that make life unbearably difficult for many people, and where sheer survival is a daily challenge. Creating better societies is everyone's responsibility.

Whatever the future holds for fibromyalgia treatment, in the present, we alone are responsible for doing what is right for us. Now in my old age,

I can afford to say "no" when something isn't in my best interest and not to care as much what others may think of me. It's too bad we have to wait till we are older to have more resilience to that central nervous system which reacts to all stimuli whether or not it is worth fussing about or not.

FMS and Medically Unexplained Symptoms (MUS)

"Open your heart to your suffering."
– Toni Bernhard

There can be little doubt that those of us with fibromyalgia or chronic fatigue syndrome have challenges that have forced us to live life differently than those who have" health privilege" (a term I am borrowing from Carolyn Thomas, dear friend and author of www.myheartsisters.org). Often thought of as malingering, hypochondriac, weak, attention-seeking, depressed people, we often live in quiet desperation. By now we recognize that we have developed these conditions because of an over-stimulated nervous system which cannot sustain itself in a healthy manner any longer.

Whatever *normal* is, our nervous system is suffering from years of responding to stimuli that are too overwhelming for our sensitive natures and has become functionally *abnormal*. In spite of the fact that fibromyalgia is not a disease, we have become chronically ill because of the pain, fatigue and myriad of other symptoms with which we are faced.

Reading the comments that were posted in the many blogs I have written over the years I am always struck by the physical and psychic pain of the readers. Some are functioning fairly well, while many others are bedridden and socially isolated. None of us live with the expectation we will be cured of the pain, fatigue, intense itching, depression, anxiety, panic, nausea, flu-like symptoms and other debilitating challenges of these syndromes. Therefore, we are left with this question posed by Toni Bernhard: "Can we live a good and fulfilling life when our activities are so severely curtailed?" The answer, of course, is yes, if we **live in the moment**. Bernhard's book *How to be Sick* is very helpful in this regard.

Her own experiences of pain are so similar to those of the many who write to me often, wondering how to keep on keeping on. After reading Bernhard's book I decided to practice her exercise which she calls "drop it," similar to "letting go." Here's how it works: As my anxieties escalate during the day, I deliberately think the thought I am having at that moment then I consciously drop it. I live with the focussed anxiety of having a flare-up from fibromyalgia and chronic fatigue, living with painful herniated disks, and worrying about having another heart attack, all the while knowing I must exercise, or at least move about, at least 30 minutes a day in spite of the pain

My fears are almost constant, but "dropping the thought" has been very helpful. I can't say the effect lasts a long time, but I have been keeping on track and repeating the phrase over and over, which is how to build new neural pathways. In short, I am taking my own advice and trying to short circuit that well-trodden anxious path and to create another by living with awareness of my habitual tendencies. I can experience joy if I live in the moment and not look back to a time I can barely remember when I did not experience pain. I can not predict what tomorrow will bring. I have only now.

A Note on Feeling Better About Visits to the Doctor

There are many of us living with "medically unexplained symptoms," such as those with post concussion syndrome, migraines, fibromyalgia and chronic fatigue, multiple chemical sensitivities, and PTSD. Most of these conditions are designated as somatization disorders, a label that can place some of us in the realm of psychiatric investigation and subsequent stigma. Working with physicians is difficult for the person with fibromyalgia as the diagnosis is often vague and the physician does not have many answers. One of the women I interviewed, Gerry, spoke about this disheartening experience: "I seldom go to the doctor now because every time I do, they say 'Well, take another pill; my clients take that pill and it helps them.' I just feel I don't want to be a guinea pig".

Toni Bernhard has wise words for those of us experiencing the added burden of not being taken seriously by the medical profession: "As you experience the unpleasant mental sensations of being treated in a dismissive manner by this medical person, instead of reacting with aversion, *consciously move your mind toward the sublime state of loving-kindness, compassion, or equanimity,* directing the sublime state at yourself."[9] This practice can help us to drop the aversion and heal our inner world.

---

[9] Bernhard, *How to be Sick,* p. 170.

Fibromyalgia and Violence

"Nonviolence means avoiding not only external physical
violence but also internal violence of spirit."
– Martin Luther King, Jr.

Violence can be defined in many ways. It is rage at its peak in the forms of shouting, yelling, hitting, rape, or any other way of inducing fear and trauma in others. Racism, sexism, homophobia, and all forms of social injustice are kinds of violence. The TV gives us a steady stream of violent situations in our own country and in places far away. It is not a kind, gentle world. We absorb violence regularly, to the detriment of our hyper-aroused nervous systems.

Because we are so sensitive, in the presence of violence or potential violence the nervous systems of those with FMS respond on high alert. If we sense even the potential for violence, we act as if it were imminent. Paradoxically, when I indulge in the guilty pleasure of reading mystery thriller novels, I find myself immersed in the inevitability of some kind of violence, but because it is fiction, the excitement quickly subsides. However, in a real-life situation I am sometimes anticipating that anger from someone else could escalate to violence and my system goes into overdrive. This is likely because my father was an explosive, angry man (although I never saw him physically harm anyone). The reality of an angry person versus the fantasy of reading about it evoke different emotions; I have not explored research which explains this phenomenon. What I do understand is that we people with fibromyalgia have a tendency to become fearful around those who are excessively angry.

The question is: how do we live in a violent world and not take on the trauma associated with it? Given our highly developed intuitive sense, we can often predict when someone is about to go into a rage and our bodies react negatively in anticipation. A simple story of someone falling, for example, can arouse in me the actual unpleasant sensation of another's pain. Hearing a racist remark can immediately bring tears to my eyes and intense anger at such injustice. Homophobic stories or jokes place me in the realm of those who are being ridiculed and my nervous system becomes highly aroused. The more dramatic forms of potential or real-life anger and violence can leave me reeling for hours or days on end.

In an article by Mark Fenske in the *Globe and Mail* [10], I found answers about how we feel another's pain. "We feel [others'] pain. Literally", he writes, describing a "class of brain cells called mirror neurons helps explain empathy and the contagious nature of emotions." Further, he writes, "these cells are thought to 'reflect' the actions and feelings of others." For that reason, among many others, it is important to reduce our own stress and avoid situations where anger and violence are common occurrences. Perhaps those mystery novels are not so good for me!

The ways in which our brains and central nervous system react to the pain of others suggests we should not be watching the terrible news these days, particularly when it documents the same hopeless issues over and over again. I don't suggest becoming ill-informed, nor lacking initiative to help overcome the droves of mis-information, or to become uninterested in the suffering of others; however, we are ill-equipped to help bring about positive change unless we change ourselves first. Taking an extended media break is good for our nervous system!

---

[10] July 7, 2011 (L6)

External Stressors: Weather, Strenuous Activity, Excitement

"Movement is a medicine for creating change in a
person's physical, emotional and mental states."
– Carol Welch

For those of us with FMS, acute pain can be brought on or exacerbated by weather changes, exercise that may only be slightly strenuous, minimal or major stress, excitement (even the good kind), viruses like colds and flus, and other physical or emotional upheavals. The list is endless.

Happily, it seems that we are on the cusp of a breakthrough in our understanding of how the nervous system processes pain. The 2021 Nobel Prize for Medicine was awarded to two American doctors, David Julius and Ardem Patapoutian, whose research has discovered receptors for temperature and touch which could pave the way for new pain-killers. Their findings show how heat, cold and mechanical stimuli affect the nervous system. Chronic pain will be addressed in a different way as a result of their research.

I am in agreement with these doctors about the importance of touch and have speculated elsewhere that our awareness of weather changes is due to our nervous system being on high alert. If only I had been a scientist and found these receptors myself! In any case, we can't control the weather but we can control our reaction to it.

For those with FMS, cold, damp or snowy weather can precipitate a flare-up of symptoms. Changes in barometric pressure are often signalled by an intense physical reaction, like the canary in a coal mine. Even strong smells can activate our nervous system. As Monica remarked, "There are times when perfumes will set me off." In fact, there are many internal or external forces at play here to bring about a trigger. For some, the trigger can cause extreme itching, intestinal upsets, extreme debilitating fatigue, emotional lability or other precursors to an acute attack. Then the acute phase of the pain sets in. We long for the weather to stabilize, hoping for a short period of respite. We prefer the chronic known pain that lives with us on a daily basis. We wish we could have refreshed sleep.

In spite of all the factors that impede us on a daily basis, as mentioned earlier, movement is a key to help us regain or at least maintain some degree of mobility and strength. This is not without many challenges. The old adages: "Rest means rust" and "If you don't use it, you lose it" are true. We must begin to *slowly* and *gently* move about to work through the steady pain and our increasing distress. It becomes a vicious cycle; pain begets more pain. To sit doing little, ruminating, is to give in to the demon that attacks us.

Without many drugs available for pain, many have found that Gabapentin (Neurontin) and Pregabalin (Lyrica) may provide some degree of relief from both acute and chronic pain. We cannot control the weather, nor can we hide from life, but there is something that can dull the pain. Nonetheless, embracing medications on a long-term basis is not without disadvantages. The longer we take a dosage, the more we need to increase it over time. The side effects of most pain medications are often numerous, like constipation, weight gain, drowsiness, dry mouth and these can be among the less serious side effects!

Do we want more new medications or do we want more emphasis on the causes that have created a huge population of those afflicted with this syndrome, so that others will not suffer as we have? Perhaps we wish for both. Finding more drugs to help with pain does not give us the answers we need. In the meantime, I wish the rain would go away!

Trauma and the Body

"The traumatic moment becomes encoded in an
abnormal form of memory, which breaks spontaneously
into consciousness, both as flashbacks during waking
states and as traumatic nightmares during sleep."
– Judith Lewis Herman

Trapped in our psyche, past traumas wind themselves into the body and present as a multitude of physical symptoms. Pain, crushing fatigue, intestinal difficulties, severe itching, rashes, tingling of limbs: the list seems endless. We seem not able to control our anxiety about when these symptoms will manifest themselves nor which kind of bodily discomfort will be next. We are constantly on guard, judging past and possible future symptoms: was this pain the same a few minutes ago? Will it become worse? If I do this or that, will it harm me? What is this new symptom about? And now, is it Covid-19?

I realize that hurt does not mean harm, but my brain does not seem to register that fact. My central nervous system is always on alert. The term "central sensitization" is now a term used more happily (or less dubiously at least) by physicians and other health care workers, so I rarely use the stigmatized word "fibromyalgia" anymore. I believe it is PTSD, but I don't mention that either. I can reflect upon my childhood and young adult life and pinpoint the traumas that etched themselves in my central nervous system. I wish the neuroscientists would ask for fibromyalgia volunteers for their PET scans and fMRIs. I would love to see these images of my brain. I know how many major traumas have affected my mind and body.

In reflecting on their own traumas, I urge those with FMS (and others!) to read Dr. Bessel van der Kolk's book *The Body Keeps the Score* from cover to cover. The book offers more evidence of the connection between our stored memories of pain and FMS flare-ups and chronic pain. Dr. van der Kolk's thesis is that after a trauma, we are left with a different nervous system than we had before the trauma, and we are left trying to control our resulting inner turmoil. He writes: "[Our] attempts to maintain control over unbearable physiological reactions can result in a whole range of physical symptoms, including fibromyalgia, chronic fatigue, and other autoimmune diseases" (p.53) (note that I do not agree that fibromyalgia is an autoimmune disease).

Dr. van der Kolk has introduced the diagnosis of Developmental Trauma Disorder in the Appendix of his book. It is a useful guide for those of us who are hypervigilant, highly sensitive, inundated with unpleasant bodily sensations, fearful and yet willing to change the brain and "befriend the body." He writes, "Being frightened means that you live in a body that is always on guard" (p.102). This is a perfect description of fibromyalgia.

One of my favourite lines in the book discusses ways to regulate our own physiology through "breathing, moving, and touching" (p.38), themes I have written about elsewhere in this book.

Finally, Dr. van der Kolk offers a hope for trauma survivors that it is indeed possible to "reconnect their thoughts with their bodies."[11]

---

[11] Review of *The Body Keeps the Score* by Dr. Stephen W. Porges (Amazon.com)

Fibromyalgia and Post-traumatic Disorders: Identical Twins?

"After a traumatic experience, the human system of
self-preservation seems to go into permanent alert, as
if the danger might return at any moment."
– Judith Lewis Herman

In an earlier section of the book, I discussed the connection between fibromyalgia and related disorders, including chronic fatigue syndrome and post-traumatic stress disorder (PTSD). I'd like to revisit the latter condition in more depth.

There has been a great deal of public awareness of late regarding PTSD. It seems as though the syndrome has become somewhat commonplace and many are quick to self-diagnose. But even more are recognizing that the condition is one caused by great stress and chronic anxiety and there are commonalities among us in our responses to traumatic experiences. What was once associated with abuse, now is believed to be the result of many possible occurrences that bring about dramatic memories, which in turn signal danger to an overly-stimulated nervous system.

It is chronic stress and subsequent chronic anxiety and flashbacks that precipitate PTSD (and fibromyalgia) since many—maybe all—people with PTSD develop fibromyalgia. What actually happens in the body is related to the interaction between 3 kinds of glands: the *hypothalamus*, which is a portion of the brain responsible for activities of the central nervous system, to the *pituitary gland* (the master gland at the base of the brain) which causes other glands to produce hormones, and the *adrenal glands*, situated on top of the kidneys, which secrete hormones that act as "chemical messengers." These three kinds of glands regulate our response to stress. The hypothalamus gives off hormones that cause the pituitary to give off another hormone and causes the adrenal to produce cortisol. When all are functioning as they should, the body is in balance; when out of balance, fibromyalgia, PTSD, and chronic fatigue occur.

But what of combat veterans who do not have PTSD or the people who have experienced a traumatic event like an accident who do not have fibromyalgia or PTSD? What is it about those of us whose psycho-social make-up affects our predisposition to these conditions? As I have repeatedly written, I believe that these "psychosomatic" (I hesitate to use this word as it conjures up bad images) syndromes are related to highly sensitive personalities. It is not necessary to speculate about whether or not a person has the predisposition to be a highly sensitive person (HSP) because of their genetically inherited qualities or because of life experiences. Nonetheless, a HSP is more likely to develop PTSD and FMS because of their personality type. It is my belief that psycho-social factors contribute to the predisposition for fibromyalgia, and a person becomes more susceptible when emotional, sexual, or physical abuse occurs.

Those with PTSD experience the same mental-emotional symptoms as those with fibromyalgia, from sleep disorders, hyper-vigilance, and panic attacks, to catastrophic thinking, a hair trigger startle reflex, flashbacks, depression, and a host of other symptoms.

What can be done to help those suffering from PTSD? The suggestions are the same as for FMS: talk and body therapy that does not include repeatedly inciting the brain to relive the trauma, relaxation techniques such as mindfulness meditation, undertaking a creative, repetitive, new-to-you hobby to change the neural pathways of the brain, movement strategies such as qi gong or tai chi, and strategies for better sleep, are among the most important. In short, it must be a mind-body approach that is undertaken that over time will change our habitual responses to everyday stressors.

Embodying Anxiety

"The truly gripping thing about anxiety had
always been how physical it was."
– Daniel Smith

I know many anxious persons who do not have fibromyalgia, but I do not know any person with fibromyalgia who does not suffer the plague of anxiety and its accompanying depression. It could be the chicken/egg dilemma, but I suspect fibromyalgia is the result of long-term anxiety which shows itself in the form of body pain, among other physical manifestations.

The book *Monkey Mind* by Daniel Smith is one in which extreme anxiety is presented honestly and sometimes overwhelmingly (with occasional sexually graphic bits). It is a sad, yet funny documentary about the many ways in which this condition can affect our bodies very dramatically.

There are many manifestations of anxiety that all of us with fibromyalgia experience: extreme fatigue, heightened startle response, hyper-vigilance, excessive worrying, sleep disturbances, nausea, racing heart, and many others, almost too numerous to list. So how do we differentiate between those which are the result of our fibromyalgia symptoms and those which are the usual signs of anxiety?

Smith talks about the differences between his anxiety, which he calls "free floating" and that of his brother Scott, whose anxiety is "somatic" (or body-based). The latter is described as "more physical," which is how I define fibromyalgia anxiety. Of his brother's condition, Daniel writes, "It starts with a twinge or an unaccustomed tightness and then rises to his mind, which, in the natural process of investigating the sensation, magnifies it, which results in further investigation, which further magnifies the sensation, creating a feedback loop" (p.26). Unfortunately, he labels this as hypochondriasis, which is not a term I am fond of because it implies that we are malingerers. Anxiety is indeed a mental health issue that is experienced as a physical disease.

The anxiety triggers we people with fibromyalgia experienced in childhood have taught us to clench and tighten our muscles, keeping our central nervous system in a state of arousal, resulting in chronic pain and subsequent fatigue along with other signs of dis-ease. Like Smith I agree that we can never be cured of anxiety, but there are strategies that will help us to address those thoughts that are going through our brains in our moments of anxiety in order to live more comfortably. While he does not use the language of mindfulness, the practice of living in the moment can help us explore what our thoughts were before the feelings of anxiety developed. In mindfulness meditation practice the mantra "thoughts are not facts" is often used. This approach to anxiety is reflected in Smith's own self-taught practice of shining a "mega- flashlight" upon his mind and asking, "[Have] I been thinking something beforehand? Was it something anxious? [Have] I spooked myself?" (p.200).

In addressing anxiety and its companion, depression, I have found the book *The Mindful Way through Depression* (authors Williams, Teasdale, Segal and Kabat-Zinn) extremely helpful. It takes the approach of cognitive behavioral therapy which has been demonstrated to be an effective non-pharmaceutical treatment for those suffering from emotional upset. I have been fortunate to have taken two separate eight-week courses in Mindfulness-Based Cognitive Therapy (MBCT) from two phenomenal therapists, and would highly recommend them. If an in-person course is not available in your area, there are courses available on-line.

Many people with FMS are on long-term disability, sick leave, fighting for benefits, and unable to afford years of therapy. However, as a group we are highly sensitive, intuitive, and generally very reflective. The simple-but-difficult MBCT-based task of exploring our own thoughts as we experience unwelcome feelings can help us along the path to self-knowledge.

In the audio recording that accompanies the *Mindful* book, author Jon Kabat-Zinn leads us through a body scan, which helps relax parts of the body affected by anxiety. If you don't have the book, you can also find several of Kabat-Zinn's guided body scan meditations on YouTube.

The daily practice of a body scan helps with the tight shoulders, stiff neck, nausea, shallow breathing, clenched jaw and other symptoms that many with fibromyalgia and chronic fatigue experience. It is more than a technique; it is a way of living with whatever state our bodies are in at the moment.

Anxiety is a plague that affects millions of people with and without FMS, but it is lifelong and constant heightened anxiety that is a clue regarding the cause of fibromyalgia and chronic fatigue. The good news is that it is possible to change our brains to address our anxiety, through discipline and repetition: there's a reason it's called mindfulness *practice*!

Symptoms on Social Media and in Film

"Trying to eradicate symptoms on the physical level can be extremely important, but there's more to healing than that; dealing with psychological, emotional and spiritual issues involved in treating sickness is equally important."
– Marianne Williamson

I have become discouraged of late with a fibromyalgia group I belong to on Facebook. One person asks about a particular symptom and others reply that they too have the symptom. While it helps to know that others are suffering to the same extent, it leaves the writer feeling helpless and a victim to the dis-ease. This is especially so when we become focused on symptoms. To be fair, sometimes there are often good suggestions as to how to deal with a particular issue, and for the most part, the group acts as a supportive community that can be very comforting. But, as we have seen, fibromyalgia is more than just a list of symptoms.

Recently I read a comment on a Facebook page about the symptom of difficulty in swallowing. This could be caused by irritation in the throat brought on by gastroesophageal reflex disease (GERD), for example. But it appears to me that when there is no known cause for difficulty swallowing, it is more commonly brought on by extreme anxiety. Difficulty in swallowing is known to be common among those who are in the midst of great stress and panic. The many symptoms of FMS and its close relatives CFS, PTSD and MCS often include shortness of breath and the sensation of a lump in the throat. The phrase "a lump in the throat" is one that brings forth an image of someone who feels extreme sadness. As during a panic attack, box breathing is helpful when having difficulty swallowing and also focussing on the five senses one at a time: what do I hear, what do I see, what is that taste, and so on. These are all safe voices for us to attend to in moments when we can't swallow our fear.

Another recent symptom posted on an FMS-related Facebook page concerns "insurmountable fatigue," in other words, chronic fatigue (or ME). This discussion thread brought mind a Netflix film I saw recently called *UNREST*, which is about chronic fatigue. As we have seen, the symptoms of CFS include physical and mental fatigue, debilitating pain, sleep dysfunction, cognitive dysfunction, sensory sensitivity, and worsening of these symptoms after even minimal exercise (so-called "post-exertional malaise"), along with a host of other physical challenges. Sound familiar, those of you diagnosed with fibromyalgia?

In all, I found the film to be very upsetting as it appeared to be focused on having a physiological cause for a condition which I believe has none. The woman portrayed in the film tried one alternative medical approach after another and it seemed as though when one new one helped as a placebo effect, she would consider herself better. Then after being bedridden for a long period of time, she would get up, walk and hike rather vigorously, and finally collapse. It was, in fact, a film which did not point out that focusing on symptoms is counterproductive. It reinforced the idea that if one can manage this particular symptom, life would resume as normal. This is a dangerous path for those of us managing many symptoms.

When it comes to living with chronic conditions like FMS and CFS, we do better when we focus on the forest, not the trees.

Flare-ups

"So, like a forgotten fire, a childhood can
always flare up again within us."
– Gaston Bachelard

A flare-up, a word for an acute attack of fibromyalgia, can be very alarming as it seems to come out of the air without warning. Even after years of living with fibromyalgia, we can become overwhelmed with an episode that we can't account for. Sometimes the flare-up is in a localized area of the body: for me, this year, it is in my hip, while last year it was in my foot. Other times it is everywhere; my nervous system is on fire and pain and fatigue run rampant throughout. For Monica, "the worst soreness is probably in my arms and my back and my legs. I find that I just have sore spots… it just feels like my skin is sore as well as the joints aching." When a flare-up happens, like many with FMS, I go through all the scenarios of the past few days and wonder what precipitated this new, intense attack.

In her book, *The Body in Pain,* Elaine Scarry writes, "Physical pain has no voice, but when at last finds a voice, it begins to tell a story." (p.3). My story, as I've told it in an earlier part of the book, included the horrors of Catholic school and believing I would die and go to hell, as well as growing up in a big city with the polio scare surrounding us. I remind myself that even though I was an anxious child with a stern, angry father and a passive mother, I no longer have that kind of trauma in my present life. I try hard to keep my life manageable, although not too restrictive. Then I remember the more important and positive thing about flare-ups: they don't last forever! They eventually subside and fade into the chronic, less debilitating fibromyalgia I have lived with for decades… until the next flare-up.

The most frightening thing about a severe flare-up is wondering if this is an unusual episode that is unrelated to fibromyalgia. Pain that brings about loud gasps, moans and outward signs of distress can be frightening to others, but even more so to myself. Is this fibromyalgia or something else I should be attending to, I wonder? If I suspect it is the same demon, I ask myself: what happened in the last few days to bring this on? It becomes easy to blame myself for excitement, overeating, or pushing myself too hard. But if the situation is beyond my control, as in a weather change, then I relax somewhat and wait for better weather conditions. After many years I no longer go to the doctor about fibromyalgia flare-ups; they have no more idea about what causes them than I do.

Living with fibromyalgia involves constant management of life events. Some days are not so painful or filled with fatigue while other days require withdrawal from life for awhile. It requires courage to pick ourselves up and start over again after an acute episode of pain.

Flare-ups come and go, and life goes on. All things considered, there are still joys to be savoured. And there is relief to be found in knowing the root cause of the flare-up and that, like a thunderstorm, it too, will pass.

Fibromyalgia Triggers

"Courage is resistance to fear, mastery of fear—not absence of fear."
– Mark Twain

A while ago, I attended a month in a chronic pain clinic. Each day we were made aware of the importance of our own minds as we lived with chronic pain. We were encouraged to use *breathing exercises* to produce enough relaxation to break the cycle of pain produced by muscle tension and allow the nervous system to relax.

Paying attention to our breathing is paramount. It is something we must do over and over again throughout the day. Research by Drs. Margaret Chesney and David Anderson at the National Institute of Health in the US found that breath holding contributes to stress-related diseases (in our case dis-eases) as our bodies become acidic; oxygen and carbon dioxide levels are then out of balance and our bodies are undermined. Those of us with anxiety need to remind ourselves to breathe deeply, as we are often shallow breathers and breath holders!

Equally as important are the *pacing strategies* we learned: breaking activities into small parts that were more manageable. Knowing, as I do, the personality patterns of those of us with fibromyalgia, I can say with certainty that we are high achievers who want to accomplish many tasks as quickly as possible. Pacing is very difficult for us. *Self-talk* was encouraged in order to practice "letting go." The motto was:" do—rest—do," finding a baseline within which we can work, stop, rest and do again. It isn't an easy task practicing these strategies on a daily, almost moment by moment basis!

In all of these daily activities it is crucial to understand the triggers that precipitate anxiety, depression, fear and a host of other emotions to which our neurons (nerves) respond with alarm. Nerves in the tissues respond to various conditions such as chemicals, mechanical issues, and temperature change. As an example, as I am writing, it has started to rain and my body has responded in a negative way, bringing on pain. It is now my responsibility to work with my mind to reassure it that we, that is my mind and body, are not in danger.

Some neurons are responsible for the danger signals that are sent to the spinal cord, and the brain decides whether or not the situation can be ignored from the danger neurons (or nociceptors). Input from the body can also send messages of danger to the brain. Muscles increase their tension and the nervous system prepares for flight with heightened vigilance. These are very simply the processes within the brain and the central nervous system that produce the many symptoms of fibromyalgia, most notably pain.

Heightened vigilance is a constant with fibromyalgia. It is raining; what does that mean to my mind? A few hours ago, the sun was shining. Is this change something the brain should be aware of? After decades of living with a hyper-aroused nervous system, my poor addled brain cannot differentiate between change that is not harmful and that which should sound an alarm. The struggle continues. Weather is a trigger for me, but I can't control the weather! I can, however, relax my brain.

Fear, the root cause of anxiety, is insidious. It wears down the physical and emotional aspects of our lives. Ailments like fibromyalgia develop from our perception of fear that is often unwarranted. The mind spins out of control and unhealthy images invade our mind, sending false messages to the brain.

The Buddhist teacher and author of *When Things Fall Apart*, Pema Chödrön, helps us to understand the triggers that perpetuate our suffering. She asks: "What is causing our pain? What would happen if we did not struggle against it?" Today, I am asking myself this question after a restless night with intense discomfort. As mentioned previously, I call my pain and anxiety "Hortense" and I speak to her regularly, saying that I understand she is trying to help me by warning me of danger, but I am really OK. I tell her to leave me alone for awhile as I need to practice my breathing. Sometimes it works. She has lived within me for almost my whole life.

After a flare-up, I can often look back and understand what the trigger has been: usually it is too much excitement or taking on more than I can handle. An excellent example of this is the holiday season. Excitement is everywhere! I can't indulge too much in all the activities or I will suffer for a few days afterwards. It is a huge trigger, yet I am drawn to the stimulation. I am drawn to helping out with the festivities. But I can learn to let others do it! I am not overly intent on being in charge.

Moderating our level of activity can help with triggering events like holidays.

Fibromyalgia and Overmedicating

"America is one of the few advanced nations that
allow direct advertising of prescription drugs."
– Robert Reich

Those of us with chronic conditions are constantly seeking relief from the myriad of symptoms that make our lives very challenging. Pain, fatigue, lack of physical abilities, sleep disturbances, depression, and rashes are but a few of the struggles which lead us to desperately seek relief in the form of medications. Living with any one of the daily distressing symptoms affects our quality of life and it is little wonder that we seek help in the form of chemicals to help us get through the day. Many, in fact, are essential to our conditions and we could not survive without them. Others are prescribed from the sheer frustration of physicians who want to help but medical answers to many perplexing conditions are not yet available to them. Such is the case with fibromyalgia. What is there to do with a patient who has chronic pain but to prescribe a pain medication that may or may not help? If the patient cannot sleep, there is a solution: sleep medication. Depression and anxiety? Medications for altering moods. The list of medications for all sorts of conditions is limitless. Pharmaceutical companies are big booming businesses whose profits know no bounds.

The recent movement to de-prescribe medications is especially relevant for those of us living with several painful and chronic conditions. However, those of us living with fibromyalgia are often used to not being listened to by health care providers. Many doctors would prefer to prescribe a pill (or several pills) to help with our ailments in spite of the fact that we are often overmedicated and highly sensitive to medications. Dr. Jaye Cohen advocates "go low [in dosage], go slow," and I am a big advocate of that philosophy.

Taking medications on a daily basis when they are necessary for life is crucial, but even then, what if the quality of life is compromised? What if, as in the case of fibromyalgia, the condition is not life-threatening? The answers to these questions are ones we have to grapple with constantly as we are the final decision- makers. Many of us have sometimes two or three serious health conditions and the medications for each conflict with one another. The pharmaceutical experiences of people with fibromyalgia are unique and there is great variation in experiences even among the community of fibro sufferers. When it comes to medications, one size does not fit all.

A review of the hundreds of comments to blog posts on my website over the years could be a rich source of data. I can attest to the vast number of anecdotal accounts of prescribed medications that have resulted in what could be called a "prescribing cascade." This occurs when a new medication is prescribed to counteract the bad effect of another.

Physicians cannot possibly remember the vast array of information that the drug reps tell them about the efficacy of all the drugs they prescribe or that they learn about online. More to the point, "new" diseases and conditions are constantly being discovered for which new drugs must be invented. Read the old: *The Medicalization of Everyday Life* by Thomas Szasz, a psychiatrist, whose work in mental illness was compulsory reading for me as a medical sociology student in graduate school many years ago.

Medications have been found to have only limited positive results in treating symptoms of fibromyalgia. Lyrica and Gabapentin have been heralded in many television commercials as the medication of choice for FMS. I have taken both in the past, but serious weight gain has been a side effect and I found that I needed to constantly increase the dosage for the medication to have any results, often with more side effects. But we are a desperate and frustrated group of people. We are willing to try almost anything, hoping for relief. For some the above-mentioned drugs are beneficial; for many, not much works.

Because I had a heart attack in 2013, I take many medications and worry about their impact on my liver and kidneys. I have decided to gradually stop taking Gabapentin regularly, except for one at night on occasion to help with nerve pain. As far as my heart medications go, I adhere to those prescriptions since they are, for the most part, evidence-based. While I worry constantly about a statin, I am searching for a medication that does not have side effects like the one prescribed for me in the hospital. I am not convinced that Gabapentin really helped me; perhaps its short-term effectiveness in my case was due to the placebo effect. Many though have found it to be helpful, and I don't want to discount their positive experiences.

Many of you, dear readers, have other chronic conditions alongside fibromyalgia. Take medications for those conditions, and if drugs for anxiety and/or depression help you, keep taking them. Many of you are poor, disenfranchised in some way, lack resources and social supports. It isn't easy living with them all. But I do have a lighthearted quote I want to share with you:

"I believe gelato is meant to be treated as medicine and taken daily as a prescription" (Betty Brandt).

FMS Plus: Living with more than one health condition

"Coping with a chronic illness is work."
– Carolyn Thomas

As mentioned in an earlier section, I am a heart attack survivor. Like many with heart disease or with a family history of heart disease, I had many questions about the leading cause of death among women. Carolyn Thomas' *A Woman's Guide to Living with Heart Disease* gave me the answers I was looking for, and better still, it is written in a style everyone can understand.

I have been following Carolyn's blog *Heart Sisters* in the eight years since my heart attack. Any questions I have had about my poor little damaged heart have been answered, not by a cardiologist, but through these blogs. Though we live thousands of miles from one another, at opposite ends of Canada, we have become friends, sort of like the penpals of yesteryear. When the American women's health collective *Our Bodies Ourselves* first decided many years ago to acknowledge 22 women in the world who had contributed to women's health, we were the only two Canadians to be so honoured. Carolyn contacted me through my website and a friendship was created. I was not particularly concerned about heart disease at the time but that was about to change. I did, however, acknowledge that fibromyalgia and heart disease had many attributes in common. Both were chronic and while one was life-threatening, the other was not. One could be treated with life-saving medications and treatments, while the other was not successfully managed with medications. More research on heart disease in general was available, (though not as much specifically for women) while fibromyalgia was still regarded by many to be malingering, especially since it appeared to affect mainly women. Both conditions are invisible and many of the symptoms are alike: pain and debilitating fatigue, dizziness, shortness of breath, and increased anxiety. Both conditions seriously affect quality of life. Heart disease is an actual disease, while fibromyalgia is a dis-ease of the central nervous system.

What has it been like for me, living with both conditions? I seem to be constantly in a state of uncertainty. I often ask myself if I am experiencing a heart symptom or an FMS flare-up? Should I see my family doctor? I don't have a cardiologist. I was told after my major heart attack and stent that I was "good to go" and unless something new developed, my family doctor could handle any concerns I had. I didn't receive any advice from cardiologists or nurses in the hospital before discharge, although I was given a pamphlet about diet and exercise. But I don't bother my family doctor about fibromyalgia issues as there isn't anything she can do. I am my own expert of this dis-ease. I would, however, book a visit with her if I was convinced it was a heart issue, but I am usually unsure, so I ruminate and wait it out.

My hip surgery, like all surgeries for those of us with fibromyalgia, was not tolerated very well, and even less so since I have heart disease. Along with aging, heart disease and fibromyalgia, I struggle with low energy. I say this with tongue in cheek however, as I have a busy and relatively happy life despite constant pain and fatigue.

I worry about the amount of exercise I get, as with heart disease exercise is primary, and I can only tolerate 20 minutes a day on my exercise bike because of FMS. Walking is what I miss the most, thanks to FMS. Overall, I would say that fibromyalgia is the most challenging in my life and heart disease, the most worrisome.

Why is it that breast cancer has gained such public sympathy and financial support, while heart disease, the leading cause of death in women, has remained a quiet torment for those of us living with (or dying from) the lack of information and treatment because we are women? Answers to these and other questions are addressed in Carolyn Thomas' blogs and her book. Carolyn and I are both white, privileged women who can speak up on our own behalf about our health issues. It is the disenfranchised, suffering people we must speak for as we walk this path with our own challenges. Neither of us see ourselves as victims, but women who have wonderful supports from family and friends. We are not poor. We live in Canada where we have universal health care. We can afford to speak out on behalf of our sisters.

PART 2

TREATING AND MANAGING FIBROMYALGIA SYMPTOMS

Mindfulness

"Peace comes from within. Do not seek it without."
– Buddha

"Breathe and let be."
– Jon Kabat-Zinn

Within the last two decades, the concept of mindfulness meditation has been adopted by schools, hospitals, businesses, police and even the military, occupations which suffer high degrees of PTSD. Who better to be taught a contemplative practice to help ease the burden of their flashbacks? Police and military personnel have jobs that are necessary to society and having resources that allow a mindful approach to their daily lives is paramount.

Empathy and compassion are integral to mindfulness meditation. It is not unique to any one religion (though often associated with Buddhism); no one "owns" this individual practice which develops our ability to listen to ourselves and to others. It can help with the current chaos and despair that permeates societies in this century with an emphasis on less aggression and anger. Mindfulness won't save the world from the many wrongdoings of the corporate world or the evils of war, but if can help address our own tendencies toward aggression and anger and cultivate peaceful societies.

The essence of mindfulness meditation is being kind to ourselves and exploring our thoughts without criticism or judgment. In his book *Wherever You Go There You Are*, mindfulness master Jon Kabat-Zinn defines mindfulness this way, "Mindfulness means paying attention in a particular way: on purpose, in the present moment, and nonjudgmentally."[12] Over time, the regular practice of mindfulness can calm our nervous systems and reduce our anxiety.

What exactly is so simple, yet so difficult about being mindful and practicing mindfulness meditation? Sitting quietly for a few minutes each day, bringing attention to our breathing, noticing our thoughts as they come and go without attaching too much importance to them—it's amazing that this practice can actually change the neural pathways of the brain. I am not diligent about daily meditation sitting, but I am getting better at reminding myself on an almost hourly basis to bring attention to my thoughts and focus at that moment on my breath.

Being mindful is practicing the art of "living in the moment"—while eating, dressing, brushing our teeth, cleaning the house, attending a meeting, playing an instrument, writing—any of the daily activities of living. Mindfulness is not just sitting quietly meditating for a few minutes each day. It is an awareness of what we are doing on a moment-by-moment basis. This is not an easy task!

Many are confused by the label of mindfulness meditation but many more are challenged by the process itself. One cannot say "There! I've meditated for twenty minutes, now I'm finished for the day." In my experience, meditation does not become easier, nor is there a "good" or a "bad" experience of the practice…it just *is*.

Thoughts are constant and practicing meditation is not to suggest that we can stop thinking. But for those of us who struggle with anxiety and rumination, meditation can be a way of looking at ourselves through a different lens. It is a way of paying attention, on purpose, moment to moment. We can learn to have self-compassion, to be non-judgmental about our thoughts and to make friends with our minds rather than struggle with challenging emotions like fear, sadness, and anger. Mindfulness meditation does not *cure* anxiety or depression. It allows us the space to not struggle against them. One should not be ashamed of either.

The chronic anxiety of fibromyalgia can be helped with a program called mindfulness-based cognitive therapy, which has been found to be extremely useful. The goal is to help the person to focus less on reacting to incoming stimuli and to accept them without judgment and without

---

[12] Kabat-Zinn, 2.

struggling against them. fMRIs have shown that practicing mindfulness meditation increases activity in the prefrontal cortex of the brain, the area responsible for good judgement and self-control. MBCT programs are a recognized treatment for people with anxiety and depression.

When "Hortense" comes to visit me, which is often, I say, "Don't come back for a few hours, ok? I will listen to you then but for now I am not ready. I need a time out." Sometimes I laugh at her as she is working hard to bring frightening thoughts to my mind. Hortense is the name of a beautiful flower. How can something as beautiful as that send me into a catastrophic thought?

For me, meditation focusses on quiet; it is about listening in for "the sound of silence". It is about *hearing* our own minds and practicing to *hear* the voices of others. (I think of these lines: "People hearing without listening" from the 1964 song "The Sound of Silence" by Paul Simon). We *hear* our minds, but we often don't listen; we need silence to do so. TVs and radios constantly blaring, phones ringing, computers and text messages being attended to almost minute by minute—none of this allows us to *hear* ourselves. Indeed, the world is filled with noise, which is a huge trigger for those of us with FMS. Quiet is soothing to our sensitive selves. Fortunately, mindfulness can be practiced anywhere, even in unquiet places like waiting rooms, on a bus, or waiting in a cashier's line.

There are many of books, journals, articles and web sites, as well as podcasts available on mindfulness meditation. Jon Kabat-Zinn's classic *Full Catastrophe Living* is a good introduction to mindfulness, as is the Mark Williams/Danny Penman book *Mindfulness: An Eight-Week Plan for Finding Peace in a Frantic World*. Tara Brach's *Radical Acceptance* also offers comforting counsel for how we can come to accept life's most challenging experiences, including chronic illness.

A common saying in mindfulness meditation is that thoughts are not facts. In chronic pain clinics we are told that hurt does not necessarily mean harm. The yoga master B.K.S Iyengar reminds us to "think light and feel light." But what are we to do when we are in a state of high arousal, waiting for disaster to fall, whether it be in the form of new FMS symptoms or the same old ones we have become accustomed to over these many years? How are we to reduce the amount of anxiety and trauma we live with everyday?

There are many strategies that we can employ, but a key one is to keep watch over our breath. Breathing is central to meditation and to living with chronic pain; slowing our breathing signals to the central nervous system that it is safe to relax. We are people who hold our breath when thoughts become fearful. Our minds need regular reassurance that the worst is not to befall us.

I have gathered some key phrases that help me calm a frightened mind. One of them is the RAW approach:

REGISTER your pain
ACCEPT it
WORK with your body, not against it.

Another method to reduce the potential threat within our nervous system is to differentiate between *emotional* and *contextual* memory. We can train our minds to bring up the specific context of the source that is calling up the traumatic information to our mind, rather than simply responding to imagined angst.

There are other strategies I have learned over the years. Here are some of the highlights:

1. Avoid catastrophic thinking. An "all or nothing" approach to life causes a lot of grief.
2. Avoid self-blaming (noticing when I am using the words "I should have…") Grant myself compassion instead of blame, as I would to a dear friend in need.
3. Avoid mind reading and imagining that the worst is about to happen. The glass is not always half empty.
4. Avoid fortune telling. The pain, fatigue, anxiety is not forever. I know that I will have some good days.
5. The pain is in the brain and can be trained to look for peace and pleasure.

In interviewing women with FMS for my first book, I was struck by how they often created their own forms of mindfulness. One of them, Bonnie, explained how she experienced moments of mindfulness in her own way: "I feel peaceful reading the Bible and sitting by myself and almost meditating. I have a little book of peaceful thoughts and I will sit alone in the dark at night when everyone else has gone to bed and just sit there and read them and think about them. That is when I feel peaceful because I have decided what's important to me"

Another woman, Sandra, spoke of her own form of mindfulness: "I try to get away by myself. I practice imagery. I just go to a relaxing place and stay there. I imagine the beauty of nature around me, waterfalls—all the little animals that are in nature."

For Rachael, another woman from the first book, who developed fibromyalgia after a car accident, tai chi helped to calm her nervous system. She also meditates for 20 minutes a day.

Mindfulness-based approaches help us to reframe our stories and challenge our responses to chronic pain. Jon Kabat-Zinn's clinic in the US and Craig Hassed's work in Australia have been successful in bringing about changes in medical curricula, so hope is building that physicians as well as other health professionals will be trained to help us help ourselves. But working with physicians is difficult for the person with fibromyalgia as the diagnosis is often vague and the physician does not have many answers.

In our meditation sessions, we can practice diaphragmatic breathing, which remains one of the most effective ways of calming our nervous system. Also known as "belly breathing," diaphragmatic breathing engages our stomach muscles and diaphragm when breathing, allowing us to effectively fill our lungs. This slow, deep breathing signals to the nervous system that it is safe to lower its guard and relax. Keeping an activity diary will help us to determine our habitual patterns; it's also a way of chronicling changes in your brain over time and will serve as a record of your own determination, as noted by Diane Jacobs.

We should not lose hope as we find ways of living with fibromyalgia. Maybe we can't cure it, but we can learn ways to avoid catastrophizing each new pain along with the old pains that never seem to leave. As Jon Kabat-Zinn notes, "Being told that you have to learn to live with pain should not be the end of the road; it should be the beginning."

Touch

"Touch is the meaning of being human."
– Andrea Dworkin

What can we do to help the empathetic, sad, and tender hearts of people with fibromyalgia? Regulating a personality that developed early in life is not an easy task. Along with psychotherapy, light exercise, and a practice of mindfulness meditation, soothing physical touch can be of great benefit to those suffering from fibromyalgia.

One of these kinds of healing touch is myofascial release, "an alternative medicine therapy claimed to be useful for treating skeletal muscle immobility and pain by relaxing contracted muscles, improving blood and lymphatic circulation, and stimulating the stretch reflex in muscles." (Wikipedia) I was intrigued by the possibility that this kind of treatment, which involves touch, might be helpful for those suffering from FMS.

Some practitioners of MFR claim that it might be able to uncover repressed memories in the receiver, as when knotted fascia begins to release, the patient begins to acknowledge painful experiences that have been stored in our memories. This interests me as I am trying to understand the relationship of past pain and the brain to help me in my day-to-day struggles with FMS.

By contrast, some argue that by uncovering painful past events, MFR creates further helplessness in the clients.

Pain scientists like Diane Jacobs focus recognize how touch affects the central nervous system. They know that it is important to help the client understand the relationship between pain and the brain rather than being a passive receiver of manual therapy. To this end, therapists like Diane Jacobs use Melzack's Neuromatrix Model, which "allows for you, the patient, to see yourself in the center of your own experience, not only part of the big picture, but *the* one who will help your own brain turn itself around."[13]

In my attempts to find relief from FMS symptoms, I have tried many touch-based treatments, including MFR, rolfing, neuromuscular massage, and other types of massages such as reflexology and jin shin. None of them have left me wanting to explore past psychological pain, although most have released tight muscle knots. Some of these forms of touch have been physically painful, while others have been soothing—none included counselling as part of the therapy. After many years of talk therapy, I have begun to realize that the stories I tell myself need to be changed. Furthermore, the ways in which I absorb the pain of others needs to be addressed. In her book *The Rejected Body: Feminist Philosophical Reflections on Disabilities*, Susan Wendell calls this "channelling other people's pain."

After my many experiences with touch-based therapies, I have come to the conclusion that while massages do soothe the body and mind, they are expensive and their effects are not long-lasting. It seems to me that if we are to deal with past experiences that have left scars in our psyche, then trained counsellors are the professionals we should seek out rather than massage therapists. Having said that I have also been reading that bringing up painful past trauma is not good for the nervous system since it reactivates it. Instead, our focus should be on working with the brain as it is today, helping it to create new neural pathways that bypass old pain. [14]

The work of such PTs as Diane Jacobs, and my own physiotherapist seem to offer me the most benefit; they advocate the use of manual therapy of the skin in an effort to gently and slowly send positive messages to the brain while simultaneously educating the client to understand the nature of pain and the benefits of physical movement. Massage therapy does indeed help with that process. Touch during Covid-19 has been challenging, but the touch professionals have found ways to care for themselves and

---

[13] See Diane Jacobs website, https://www.dermoneuromodulation.com

[14] For a very comprehensive understanding of the mind/brain that is much easier to understand than most of what is written by those whose research is focused on consciousness, please read *The Biology of Mind: Origins and Structures of Mind, Brain and Consciousness* by Deric Bownds.

others during this epidemic and we must have the courage to allow them to touch us.

We can't undo the life traumas that have affected our nervous systems and our lives, but we can try to understand how we are not completely helpless and doomed to a life without hope. We do not have to care about other people's happiness to the exclusion of our own healthy mind set. We are not personally responsible for everybody else's happiness or pain; being in that head space absolves others from caring for themselves. It is foolhardy to believe we can solve other people's problems. This is our daily challenge and great opportunity for healing ourselves.

Minimizing Our Anxiety

"When anxious people anticipate something bad about to
happen—such as being confronted with creepy pictures of snakes
or spiders— their right frontal insulas go into overdrive."
– Blakeslee and Blakeslee

Many of us with fibromyalgia can remember childhood as the beginning of a lifetime of fear and anxiety. Since there might have been a significant childhood episode that triggered this dis-ease called fibromyalgia, it stayed with us while other troublesome events in our lives piled anxious feelings one on top of the other. It is as if we have accumulated and stored anxieties in our psyche until we can't differentiate between everyday events that aren't fearful and those that are. We feel things too deeply. Our empathy capacity is filled to overload. We cannot respond healthily to any form of drama or excitement.

While we may experience some of the warning signs of FMS in childhood, such as fainting, hyperventilating, or panic attacks, it appears as though we are usually able to live a normal life until a major crisis precipitates full-blown fibromyalgia, generally in early middle age.

Understanding our triggers is especially helpful. In *The Body Has a Mind of Its Own*, Sandra and Matthew Blakeslee write about how "your brain is teeming with body maps—maps of your body's surface, its musculature, its intentions, its potential for action, even a map that automatically tracks and emulates the actions and intentions of other people around you" (p.11). Given that we respond not only to our own feelings and moods, but also those of others, it is little wonder that we are acutely aware at all times about what is going on in the world around us, which can often be overwhelming.

Consider an alternative: rather than focusing on the dreadful news of the day and the despair of so many who are suffering, should we not focus for a few brief moments on the beauty of the seasons, being grateful for the good things in our lives, and the joy of just being alive in this moment? Being fraught over the difficulties of our lives and the state of the world should not cloud the joy that is around us. In the words of Patty, one of the women I interviewed all those years ago, "I try to keep my spirits up. I'm an outgoing person anyway. I try not to let [fibromyalgia] destroy me because no matter what stress I've had in my life I still try to keep a smile."

Befriending Change

"When you're finished changing, you're finished."
– Benjamin Franklin

Many people report their fibromyalgia began with an accident, surgery, violence or another episodic event that was physically shocking to the nervous system. Some medical professionals call this "primary fibromyalgia." However, fewer report that major life changes like marriage, parenthood, divorce, job loss or change, loss of loved ones, chronic illness, widowhood, moves, menopause, retirement, even significant birthdays can be equally as traumatic to the nervous system. These events often precipitate what's known as "secondary fibromyalgia"; other risk factors include living with homophobia, racism, disabilities, and poverty.

Adjusting to a new life circumstance is often not easy even for those not suffering from FMS. Uncertainty about the new transition develops, and for the person with fibromyalgia or prone to it, anxiety brings about hyper-arousal of the nervous system, coming from a fear of the unknown. Instead of catastrophizing what the new life circumstance might bring, we should be open to seeing the new with a degree of promise and hope. It's about seeing the rainbow somewhere on the horizon, even if there is grief, pain and sadness associated with the change.

It is a good exercise for us to record all the major transitions we have experienced during our lifetimes and how we processed them in our minds. Some were accompanied by joy and hope while others became associated with fear, grief and panic. Some transitions involved mixed emotions. Understanding how our brain led us down a certain path will result in insights into what led to fibromyalgia. A good therapist can help; talk therapy for a period of time cannot be underestimated. Through studying the past, we learn our future.

One woman I interviewed, Jill, had a standing appointment with her psychiatrist with whom she had a good relationship. "I see a psychiatrist and I have been seeing him for the last seven years because my doctor… doesn't seem to know a lot about fibromyalgia and I really get the feeling that he's not all that interested in learning about it." Having a psychiatrist who was willing to find information and help her through her past traumas was very important for her well being; in her words, "I don't know what I would do without my psychiatrist. I truly don't."

Fibromyalgia and Male Caregiving

"Caring is pivotal to keeping the human enterprise going, yet its
function is invisible in the organization of our daily lives."
– Sheila Neysmith

In my first book I discussed the issue of caregiving with the women
living with fibromyalgia, asking who were the people who supported them.
Their answers often surprised me. I am one of the fortunate ones who has a
partner with a caring nature. He is my biggest supporter and without him I
don't know how I would survive the pain and fatigue. I generally feel guilty
about the limitations of my life and how they have impacted his. It can't be
easy since those of us with fibromyalgia usually look healthy, and even the
caregiver must wonder at times if we really are suffering as much as we say
we are. The irony of all this is that people with fibromyalgia are often in a
state of hyperarousal of the nervous system because they themselves were
once super-carers of others! Furthermore, the guilt we experience because
others are taking care of many of our needs is a conundrum we are forced
to live with. But allowing others who are willing to care for us, especially
during flare-ups, is something we must accept. Even though our condition
is invisible, others who love us– our spouses, family, and friends— can be
invaluable.

Before I retired from my life as a university professor, I supervised
several graduate students who wrote their theses about the caregiving
strain on women who were caring for elderly parents. I knew all the
symptoms: exhaustion, lack of support, resentment, guilt, limited time
for oneself and so on, but the research was generally about women in the
sandwich generation, caring for elderly parents while also caring for their
own children. I now find myself in a reverse position of living with a man

who is the primary caregiver in our home. I can watch my spouse firsthand and see much of the invisible work he does as a carer. I am constantly wondering what he must be feeling when he hears another complaint from me about having a bad day, my frequent bouts of hopelessness, my groans of pain and sleepless nights. I feel guilt when I can't go walking with him, or do my share of housework, or have travel insecurities and worries that I can't control since they are based upon my own loss of control. I know how fortunate I am to have such wonderful support and my heart goes out to those without it, going it alone on this challenging journey.

Many caregivers suffer in silence and worry privately about the fate of their loved ones. One such person is Maurice Clarke, who served as secretary of the Rugby (UK) Fibromyalgia Support Group, and once ran a website for male caregivers called *FibroLads Care.* I asked to interview him regarding his own caregiving role in the home since his wife has fibromyalgia (his wife has kindly agreed to allow him to share his feelings with us publicly.) I asked Maurice what inspired him and his wife to begin a support group for spouses of women with fibromyalgia.

Here is part of his reply:

"She and I started our support group due to experiences in the Midlands and Norfolk (UK) in attending other support groups as members and then finding none in our own area. We had travelled some 20 miles to attend another group which eventually folded due to lack of support.

I had good PR experience so was able to get a lot of free local articles on the new group and we grew that way.

The group is for men – I spoke to several women members about their partners attending and they thought it was a great idea but they [women] did not see any value in attending. Men generally do NOT like talking about their feelings, whereas women are freer in this regard.

My wife and I see and have contact with 30 or more regular people with FM most with partners – ranging from 25 to 80 in age. Some are still working and overall, in varying degrees of pain. Most have other issues with the FM which makes treatment hard."

Maurice said that the group usually met in a pub, where between 5 and 10 men would sit around a table and share stories about their lives as caregivers for their partners. He said that the workload associated with running the group was hard on him and his wife, especially as attendance was often spotty.

Still, according to Maurice, "Many of our long-established members who are loyal have become more outgoing and friendly and to them the group has been a life saver."

In keeping with what Maurice said about the difficulties of being married to someone with FMS, one of the women I interviewed for my first book, Gerry, spoke about the strain her condition placed on her own marriage: "My husband and I used to walk on Sunday all around Stanley Park. We just love to walk; we like to swim. My husband just can't understand [my fatigue]". FMS-related fatigue is not just being tired; it is a crushing symptom that sometimes makes even walking around the house an overwhelming task. This is very difficult for anyone to understand as the condition is invisible; if we had a broken arm, our cast would show others that we are unable to function in certain ways.

It's important for caregivers, male or female, to allow themselves to feel what they are feeling without guilt. If there is a support group in your area for men who become caregivers, consider joining it and talk about your challenges. And please try to understand when you become a caregiver that life with fibromyalgia is not easy for either of you.

Women and Caregiving

"It is possible to move through the drama of our lives without
believing so earnestly in the character that we play."
– Pema Chodron

I have been a caregiver for most of my life as a mother, a nurse, and caregiver to elderly parents, and it has taken a toll on me in many ways. How do I learn to set boundaries and stick to them? What makes me think that I can *mother* the world? Isn't that a kind of self-sacrificing arrogance? What is it that prevents many of us from changing our thoughts, emotions, and ways of being in the world even when we know that what we are doing is harmful to our health?

When I was a professor teaching courses in gerontology, I supervised several graduate students who did research with adults who were caregivers for older parents. Their stories were filled with issues of guilt, burn-out, worry, fatigue, anger, hopelessness, often love, but also intense dislike of the parent. Generally, women were the caregivers and because they had busy lives of their own, they were overwhelmed with responsibilities. I taught these courses in elder issues, never really thinking that they would someday become my own dilemma as I coped with the demands of 90+ year old parents. My father suffered from borderline personality disorder, and he initiated drama and crises everywhere he went. While dealing with the pain and fatigue of fibromyalgia, then a heart attack, I also cared for him and my anxious mother.

Speaking about the burden faced by female caregivers in his book *The Making of an Elder Culture*, Theodore Roszak writes: "It is women-daughters or daughters-in-law-far more than men who are suffering the pressure of home-based caregiving. While caregivers come in many shapes and sizes, their gender is all but uniform" (p. 99-100). It is also true that the majority of people who suffer from "caregiving fibromyalgia" are women. Combining caregiving and fibromyalgia often results in social, physical and psychological crises for the caregiver as well as the recipient of care.

Of course, as we have seen, women are not the only caregivers. I know of many men who are the providers of care and suffer from caregiving strain. It has been noted that the kinds of care that women and men give to those who rely on them differ rather dramatically. Practical support seems to be the most common kind of caregiving among men, while emotional work is added to practical tasks among women.

Caring for a parent, spouse or a child with disabilities carries with it a range of emotions, along with both physical and psychological demands. For me, the challenges were those of elderly parents and the strain on my emotions as I tried to appease, organize, placate and give support within relationships that were fraught with difficulties. I had difficulty setting boundaries and caring for myself along with my parents. The Harvard Medical School booklet *HEALTHbeat* discusses "the power of self compassion," pointing out that self-compassion (or self-care) is a learnable skill. Without it our mood is not friendly, either towards ourselves or the world at large.

Many have written to me of the difficulties of living with fibromyalgia plus the responsibilities of caring for a family member. In particular, much of this correspondence has been from mothers caring for disabled children. I often think of those who suggest kindly that support groups would help. However, they often fail to take into consideration that this is a time commitment that many can ill afford. Women's lives are often shaped by their commitments to others, and sometimes unwanted responsibilities, often to the detriment of our own needs.

As difficult as it may be, taking time to care for ourselves as well as others is essential.

Not Giving Ourselves Away

"Self development is a higher duty than self sacrifice."
– Elizabeth Cady Stanton

As I read more and more about brain mapping and how to change the pain mappings in my brain, I am reminded about how often I have written about the ultra sensitive person. This is the "empath," the person who senses what other people are feeling and takes on the emotions of others as though they were her/his own (I don't mean this in the usual sense of the psychic person, or in any mystical way). I still stand by that description of the person with fibromyalgia. We are like a toxic sponge! This type of person is often self-sacrificing and doing good for others, what Dr. James Rochelle calls "goodism." My physiotherapist calls this "giving yourself away." FMS sufferer Florence Nightingale is a prime example of this kind of self- sacrificing behaviour.

When we aren't getting our needs met, we are subject to repressed anger, among other negative emotions. Often the result is trying harder to please in an effort to be pleased ourselves. Why is it that Christianity and other religions value doing for others to the point of giving more to them than to oneself? This cannot be the essence of good health for those with chronic invisible dis-eases. If we don't understand ourselves and our frequent neglect of our own bodies and brains, it stands to reason we (and others) will suffer in some way. So, what is the answer? Certainly not to become self-absorbed or do nothing for others. But how about we connect with ourselves first?

The ultra-sensitive person who is keenly attuned to the needs of others becomes almost immune to what she desires for herself. Anxiety becomes a way of life. If we do not meet everyone's needs, we believe we are less than perfect. Fear, anger, anxiety and other negative responses inhibit us from healthy self-expression and the brain is always on guard, on duty. We cannot meet what **we** perceive to be others' unrealistic expectations of us. How can we ever be that perfect person and why are we so hard on ourselves?

The unconscious part of our brains stores repressed, unpleasant emotions, including past traumas, both physical and emotional, and this part becomes overcrowded with negativity, leading to FMS symptoms like pain and fatigue. If we continue to treat the symptoms but not the root cause of these emotions, we are giving ourselves away even more. It is little wonder that after a surgery, an episode of emotional or physical abuse, an accident, or prolonged trauma of some kind, those with fibromyalgia tendencies will have reached the tipping point in our already overstimulated nervous system. Full blown fibromyalgia and chronic fatigue ensue.

We now understand and accept that the brain is changing all the time and that we can change those maps that are not helpful to us and develop alternate pathways. In other words, the brain is not hardwired, nor static. The new brain science is becoming increasingly fascinating! Psycho-neurologists are the professionals who can assist us with this process, not rheumatologists. In particular it must be noted that physicians know very little about fibromyalgia. Neuroscientists' work is changing the way we view the brain and it is to be hoped that their work will soon turn more specifically to the increasing numbers of people suffering from fibromyalgia.

Some of the practical work that has been successful in this regard is that done by those who write about trauma which can over-arouse our nervous system. At her website, http://www.myshrink.com, Dr. Suzanne LaCombe writes about Self-Regulation Therapy as a psychotherapy approach "that is based on [our] innate ability to regulate arousal." While this and other books or sites I reference are not specifically about fibromyalgia, I have included them as fitting in with the points I am making about the hyperarousal of the nervous system.

I have read of a group of women with FMS, chronic fatigue and multiple chemical sensitivities who get together in Toronto as a reading group to discuss wellness. This activity ties into the perspective of remapping the brain to focus on positive and creative input and ideas rather than triggering the old negative emotions that bring about flare-ups. Such positive gatherings with friends and peers help to create alternate neural pathways. Perhaps this is why prolonged talk therapy has not been helpful for people with fibromyalgia. Reliving past injuries of a physical or emotional nature only reactivates the nervous system. Instead, it is more important to recognize our reactions rather than the specific events related to the trauma.

In his book *Waking the Tiger,* Dr. Peter Levine writes that we should become unattached to our symptoms to reduce the power they have over our minds: "We need to release them from our minds and hearts along with the energy that is locked in our nervous systems" (218).

I urge my readers to delve into the book by Norman Doidge, *The Brain that Changes Itself.* I have watched him on television where he discusses the new advances in neuroscience and points out how the brain is changing all the time and even more so when innovation is introduced. Groups getting together in a positive way is one very effective means of remapping unpleasant memories in the unconscious part of our brains, and is one form of self-care. As Diane Jacobs has told me, "neuroplasticity is your friend."

We don't need to give ourselves away without attending to ourselves. Tapering off this habit is difficult for many of us to do and it takes a long time. Being the perfect woman exhausts and depletes both our body and brain. Why do we continue to take on someone else's problems as well as our own?

There are strategies to help bring about self-compassion. Among them: Comfort your body, including healing touch by you or someone else; write a letter to yourself, forgiving yourself for memories that bring about shame, perceived or real; give yourself encouragement; practice mindfulness frequently during the day.

Embracing Change

"The changed brain stays changed."
– Barbara Arrowsmith-Young

Fibromyalgia is a syndrome with a constellation of symptoms that are often used to define us. There are pitfalls in this kind of stereotyping that can become stigmatizing. Even worse, a person with a label can use their condition to explain away specific behaviours that the person identifies with as essential personality traits. How often have we heard someone say, "Well, that's just the way I am. I can't change"? In fact, we can change, as emerging neuroscience is discovering.

A thought-provoking book in this regard is *The Woman who Changed her Brain* by Barbara Arrowsmith-Young and although not about fibromyalgia, it relates to how we can change old neural pathways in the brain. Her focus is on neuroplasticity and how to bypass what neuroscientists call "traffic jams in the brain," (a fitting term for those of us with FMS!) Arrowsmith-Young has shown that although she was born with a brain that presented many challenges and caused her to be labelled a learning-disabled child, she was able to change her old neural pathways and overcome her dis-ability. She addresses the topic of neurodiversity and how no two people share the exact same brain map: "Neuroscience holds great promise in that it offers insight into the differences between us and the different ways that each of us thinks, learns, processes information, and responds emotionally—all of which are determined in no small part by the singular makeup of our brains. And with an understanding of the plastic nature of the brain, we can harness this property to positively change its functioning" (36).

Labels are often more dangerous than they are helpful when we identify with the condition they describe, making it a core part of our identity. With

137

the constant pain of FMS, we often understandably experience depression and the fear that the pain will never subside. Is being labelled a *depressive* useful? We do have the characteristics of being highly sensitive and overly empathetic; do those labels help or hinder us? Do we need support groups that often enhance our feelings of being different and unique? Have we psychologized ourselves into categories to the extent that we resist change? The world may not be as we have seen it in the past and that is a frightening thought, sending our amygdala into its usual tailspin.

Language is a powerful force and the ways in which physical conditions are written or spoken about have the ability to either motivate us or condemn us to acceptance of the status quo. I recently asked a therapist to help me with the language of chronic pain. How can we find words that are less solidified and less hopeless? She suggested "pain that is stuck", which implies that it is possible to *unstick*. So, I can now say, "I don't have 'chronic' pain; I have symptoms that are stuck in the brain and I am working to release them." Still, I am stuck for words to describe FMS and on the look out for language that will unite us, rather than label us negatively.

One of the women I interviewed, Deb, described those of us with fibromyalgia as those who persevere: "The people with these types of personalities— we pursue [information], we don't give up, like I haven't given up yet. I've been diagnosed with it, but it doesn't have me".

Living Our Best Life

"Courage is resistance to fear, mastery of fear, not absence of fear."
– Mark Twain

With all the chaos and disasters being reported hourly in the news, it is essential for those with sensitive nervous systems to go on regular media diets. While we can't hide in isolation from outside influences, we need to be mindful of what we are feeding our brains, just as we are aware of what we feel like when we have eaten a lot of junk food.

Just as in the general population, those with fibromyalgia display different personality traits. Many of us are introverts, craving peace and quiet while still needing to be around people on our own terms. Others are extroverts while at the same time easily over-stimulated. But we all have in common our anxiety, hyper-vigilance, and an overly empathetic, highly sensitive nature. For those reasons we are sensitive to injustice, so often on display in the news. We are intuitive about the good and the bad in others and quick to judge ourselves, particularly if we believe we are not courageous. People with fibromyalgia are emotionally contagious to the pain of others. We live in fear we will be found lacking in strength of character, deriding ourselves over even mentioning our chronic symptoms of pain and fatigue. We appear "normal" and most cannot sense our pain.

Living with a chronic disorder usually changes our lifestyle and abilities. While in my previous life I was "out there" fighting for issues of social justice: women's rights, LGBTQ+2 issues, race, labour and workers' groups, and attending climate change demonstrations, I can no longer call up the energy, nor do I have the physical ability to participate in social activism. Within these marginalized groups of people, I would find kindred spirits as they too would no doubt suffer from fibromyalgia in great numbers. I must leave the struggles to the younger generation, one that will face more challenges than ever. My thoughts go to my grandchildren and the chaos and fears they have inherited.

Happiness isn't a natural state for me. I admit that I don't trust it. My fury at injustice must be turned to gentleness towards myself and I must work to try to stop imagining the darkest possible scenario. Currently during Covid-19, the volume in my central nervous system is turned up high and hope is not an easy thing to develop. Still, I watch those younger and more fit people who are resisting injustice and I want to believe in something better, to imagine a more hopeful world. Those who are marching for climate change, Black Lives Matter, All Children Matter, LGBTQ2+ rights have the power to bring about a better future. There is indeed hope for the world.

Quieting Our Noisy Brains

"Our memory is in large part the starting point for how we think,
how our preferences form, and how we make decisions."
– Maria Konnikova

Some time ago on CBC radio, I heard an interview with Dr. Maria Konnikova regarding the science of memory and became intrigued with the ways in which she has based an understanding of neuroscience upon the brains and memories of two fictional characters: Sherlock Holmes and Dr. Watson. in her book *Mastermind*. Being a Holmes lover and extremely interested in how the brain works, I hastened to read Konnikova's amazing book *Mastermind* regarding these two distinct minds, each of which contains something she terms the "brain attic." This term she borrows from Holmes himself, who said: "I consider a man's [sic] brain originally is like a little empty attic, and you have to stock it with such furniture as you choose" (cited in Konnikova, 26).

I have often referred to my own brain as one which is full of memories and needs emptying. In that, I am similar to the Watson attic, which is constantly on high alert, and is, in Konnikova's words, "jumbled, largely mindless" (29) and needs cleaning out. We need our brain attic to be more selective and observant in its choice of memories to store and recognize the ones which precipitate anxiety.

By contrast, the Holmes attic is deliberately furnished with a more curated selection of memories, ones that keep the brain in its thinking place rather than being hijacked by the fight or flight response of the triggered amygdala.

Konnikova emphasizes the importance of meditation training as a way of clearing out the brain attic memories, although as she says, it takes "practice, practice, practice." I would remind readers that, while this is not a book about fibromyalgia, it does contain valuable lessons on how to train the brain to remain calm so we can use our problem-solving abilities rather than simply responding to crises.

Those interested in emptying their own cluttered brain attics may want to know how things got so bad in the first place! A person with high anxiety has stored long-term anxiety-provoking memories in the brain attic's "storage space" which Dr. Konnikova points out is called **consolidation**. It is likely that childhood trauma has been responsible for this storage. Every time a new stressful event occurs, the "file" (as Konnikova calls it) is pulled out and more is added to the memory file. When this happens, the attic becomes more cluttered. It is at this point that we often develop brain fog and our thoughts become less than coherent. Often, we say the wrong words or forget simple ones (as happens in old age, as I am discovering!) This highly anxious person's fight-or- flight Watson brain is on the lookout for ever more anxious memories to add to the file since our brains are hardwired to search for—and find—patterns. It does not discriminate.

The body of the anxious person is also affected by the constant addition of new material to the anxiety file. Body systems which are affected include the muscular-skeletal system, the immune system, and the digestive system, causing more anxiety to add to the memory pile up.

In his book *Fibromyalgia Relief,* Lars Clausen also writes of ways to unpack the cluttered attics that cause us anxiety and other painful FMS symptoms through a process called "memory reconsolidation." He says, "Unless we reconsolidate the emotions we have of our past memories, we will continue reacting to the old emotion of each memory" (p.71). Consolidation is considered to take place within the first few hours of the event being remembered, so it is necessary to consciously stop these emotions from becoming part of the furniture of the attic! Not all neuroscientists are in favour of reconsolidation, but there are those who suggest that previous memories can be changed through reactivation of the memory.

Konnikova advocates being mindful, but there is more to changing the brain and subsequently those unwelcome stored memories. The vast scientific literature that has been presented over the past few decades based upon the neuroplasticity of the brain points to other techniques as well as learning to observe our mental patterns. Movement such as Qi-gong, yoga, NIA dance, taking on new tasks that are creative and repetitive, music, and art all feed into the realm of strategies that together can activate new pathways. Good sleep and healthy food are paramount. Our goal in doing this is to develop a Holmes brain where "thoughts, properly filtered, can no longer slyly influence your behavior without your knowledge," (Konnikova, 21).

Pulling Ourselves Up by Our Bootstraps

"We have a lot of anxieties, and one cancels out another very often."
– Winston Churchill

Many of us can trace our anxiety back to our childhoods. I have spoken about some of my own back story in an earlier section of this book, along with a childhood that featured anxious parenting, Catholic nuns who terrified me with thoughts of hell, and a move from a large city to a small town as an adolescent. This was followed by the beginning of my life as a nurse; like the other students, I was used as a source of free labour in a diploma-based nursing school. Other stressors in my life included nursing in general, an early bad marriage, three C-sections, a divorce, completing a PhD as a single parent, being stalked, a remarriage with a blended family of five teenagers, caring for elderly parents, and finally a heart attack, followed by a hip replacement. Now, of course, aging has reared its challenging head and Covid. Each new crisis, no matter the seriousness, triggers the amygdala.

One might look at this list and believe it is not as horrific as the lives of those who suffer greater atrocities, for example people in the Ukraine. More locally the First Nations children who were forced into Catholic schools, taken from their parents and whose graves have recently been found in Canada. The survivors of these atrocities have stored memories which haunt them daily.

I have a roof over my head, am not financially downtrodden, and have a supportive mate and friends. It would seem that I could reason my stresses away. Nonetheless, there are two kinds of people: those who thrive in acute stress situations and are resilient and those who don't feel there is any strength left to overcome even minor stressful life events.

Beginning life as a high-energy person, I am no longer the woman I once was when I felt I could conquer the world. I am very self-conscious about discussing my FMS symptoms with most people, especially a certain friend who suffers from what I call "boot-strap-ism." She believes one should just get on with life and that aging is not a state of gloom and doom; she often mentions old star performers as an example of embracing old age. Perhaps I too should do the same, uncurl those bootstraps. After all, the alternative to old age is not all that desirable! I do try, then a flare-up occurs, often for no reason that I can identify, and I simply cannot pull myself away from anxiety. Is it another heart attack, I wonder, even now after nine years have passed?

I cannot feel too sorry for myself. I am a privileged woman. I have not suffered the ravages of war, racism, extreme poverty or homophobia. As young women we are trained for fear, but many of us become strong, fearless, resilient women as we age. Others struggle with a hyper-aroused central nervous system that produces a highly vigilant woman (or man) who is overly empathetic and lives with fibromyalgia, chronic fatigue, and PTSD. We can't judge another's fears and anxieties. We can never know the struggles someone else goes through. Self- compassion is paramount, rather than self- criticism.

It doesn't help to know that many are suffering from mental anguish at the state of the world so our attempts to cultivate hope for the future may seem far- fetched. But without trying to seem artificial, we can find small things to smile about several times a day and only hope that our children and grandchildren will profit from our mistakes. Accessing mental health therapy if it can be afforded, writing gratitude journals, living in the moment, and taking care of ourselves seems to be the only alternatives to complete feelings of doom.

The Roller Coaster of Emotions

"You gain strength, courage, and confidence by every experience
in which you really stop to look fear in the face."
– Eleanor Roosevelt

Those of us with FMS are generally very hard on ourselves, believing we are hypochondriacs and malingerers. I often call myself whiny and have to pay attention to what I am telling my brain that reinforces negative feelings about the kind of person I am. I give in to fear if I don't give myself a message to stop. Monica also speaks of the runaway negative emotions that accompany FMS: "Sometimes I feel like I'm in some kind of emotional roller coaster and I have to really stop and think, you know, what I'm reacting to…. Is it just something within myself or is it really this major? Like I'm constantly questioning, you know, whether I'm blowing things out of proportion or whether I'm actually seeing things in reality because I don't really know." Not knowing in itself causes fear.

In an article entitled "Face Fear and Keep Going,"[15] Carolyn Gimian writes, "Fear, while critically necessary for life itself, can be horrifying and crippling. It can also eat away at us day in and day out" (59). Those of us with FMS are full of fears: What if we become completely disabled? What if this pain never stops? What if we become housebound?

Many of us with FMS may have sought relief from our fear-causing symptoms at pain clinics, though several of the participants in the month-long class I attended said their pain was much worse after the constant reminder of living with chronic pain! Their fears worsened as they listened to stories of others whose pain seemed different from theirs: If it was more,

[15] *Mindful* magazine, April 2016

they wondered if they would become as bad as the ones who seemed to be suffering intensely, and if it was less, they still wondered if they were in more danger as time went on. The brain and its neural networks are relentless in their desire to protect us from real or perceived danger. For those of us with fibromyalgia it is a heightened interweaving of various components of the brain dwelling on fearful possibilities.

But there are solutions to turning down the volume in this noisy brain of ours. I have quoted Dr. Norman Doidge and his book *The Brain That Changes Itself,* as he writes about how the brain is not rigid but has adaptive abilities. Among many of his suggestions is the simple act of conscious walking, or using music and voice to stimulate brain circuits, or touch therapy, among other ways of changing the brain. Those of you who have practiced meditation have no doubt been part of walking meditation practices. The brain can heal itself and it can find new ways of taming those neurons that are so quick to send messages of fear and anxiety through a conscious plan to bring about change. Exercise of any kind, which need not be vigorous, just even movement, is a beginning process for those of us with a desire to experience peace. Our racing minds can be tamed with even a simple practice: take a one-minute mindful pause or step several times a day. Take many short breaks a day to practice deep breathing.

Allowing Our Emotions

"Having that sense of anger leads people to actually feel some
power in what otherwise is a maddening situation."
– Jennifer Lerner

There can be little doubt that emotions play a large part in a
fibromyalgia flare-up. The emotions can be happy, sad, fearful, anxious
or any of the myriad of other feelings which affect us throughout the day.

In an article in the *Globe and Mail*[16] written by Sarah Barmak, it is said
that the study of emotions "is now among the hottest areas of academics."
Barmak has cited the YouTube series of Yale University's June Gruber
called *Experts in Emotion.* I can read and watch this academic research
and understand it theoretically, meditate, live in the moment, exercise;
still, my emotions are becoming more powerful and less able to control
than they once were. I willingly allow myself to turn my anxiety into anger
and quite frankly, it feels good! I can tell myself not to judge and become
self-critical, to accept that these are passing emotions, not hard and fast
facts and push them gently aside, but this past two years of Covid-19 and
too much reflective thinking has resulted in complex emotions that have
been flooding through my body and brain and are often overwhelming.
As women we often supress our anger; I no longer want to.

For me, the most intense emotion I experience these days is what I call
justifiable anger: I am angry that I have lived and continue to live with
daily pain and fatigue. I cannot remember a time in my life since I was 25
that I have not experienced pain in one form or another. Now, with aging I
find that the pain is not subsiding despite all that I do. I have osteoarthritis

---

[16] July 27, 2013, *Focus*, 3.

of the hips and degenerative disc disease as do most people my age. What has made me the angriest is the newer challenge of living with heart disease and aging. These are not the golden years. When people tell me I look well, I cannot tell them the truth: most days I feel unwell. I cannot differentiate between the symptoms of aging, fibromyalgia and heart disease. I have fatigue from all three (and probably from medications). I am taking medications for my circulatory system while my central nervous system is on fire.

People will understand when I say I have had a heart attack but not if I say I have fibromyalgia. After all these years, fibromyalgia is highly disregarded; that is, the emotion I am feeling about this syndrome: anger. I am angry because women and heart disease is an issue that has scarcely been addressed, except from a few notables like expert Carolyn Thomas at her website, www.myheartsisters.org.

When I was a child there was a children's radio program called *Maggie Muggins* which always ended with the saying: "I don't know what I'll do tomorrow." In fact, the same can be said for my emotions these days: I don't know what I'll feel tomorrow, but I can be sure the emotions will be passionate. But for now, I must try to live in the moment. Perhaps this passion is not all negative; it might just be a survival tactic. There is after all, justifiable anger. So far, I have not shown this emotion but kept on with that stony smile. I hope to burst open some day, but in a controlled fashion after I have learned not to become angry at myself in the process.

Dressing for Comfort

"I base most of my fashion sense on what doesn't itch."
– Gilda Radner

There isn't anything more comforting to me than cloth that is soft and soothing. Mostly, it is cotton that gives me a feeling of being in a cocoon. The itching brought on by FMS has made comfortable fabric even more of a priority in my life. Fabric also gave me the basis for a new creative interest: quilting.

Many years ago, in an effort to "change my brain" regarding pain, I followed the advice of experts and took on a project which was creative and new to me. In addition, it is somewhat repetitive, also part of the triad of characteristics that make up this endeavor. Quilting was my hobby of choice; because I had never sewed before, it was indeed a steep learning curve, but it brought me into the realm of fabrics.

I found myself in shops that were new to me as I walked among the bolts of material that were either comforting or irritating to the touch. It was then that I finally understood why I have never been a fashion queen. Fashion has never been interesting to me. I am only at ease in soft, cotton fabrics, otherwise my body is "itchy and scratchy." Rashes, tingling, burning will develop if the clothing I wear is not soothing to touch.

When my oldest son was a toddler, he would take a piece of new clothing and rub it against his face, and if he did not like the feel of it, he would say it was "picky" and would not wear it. It seems as though his sensitivity to fabric was hereditary! Raised in the 1970s, he and his two brothers were a product of those terrible acrylic, scratchy clothes for boys. Nylon, rayon and other non-natural fabrics were the bane of their existence.

Raised in the 1950s myself, I remember the unpleasant sensations of crinoline skirts, tight waistbands, itchy dresses and uncomfortable high-heeled shoes. I would itch after wearing a crinoline and anything tight, in particular nylon stockings and later pantyhose.

I am certain that all the itching and subsequent skin problems that we fibromyalgia persons experience is no doubt exacerbated by irritating fabric against the skin, make-up that is poisonous, and shoes that affect our feet in later life. Is it little wonder that more women than men experience itching and scratching until the skin erupts? Added to which is the pressure women are under to dress fashionably, which usually means uncomfortably.

The fashion industry is the second greatest polluter of the environment after oil. Not only is it responsible for pollution of the earth, but it also pollutes our sensitive bodies. Do try a day without makeup and nail polish; poisonous substances have been found in nail polish that can affect the endocrine system and potentially the reproductive system. Spend a week in soft, loose, non-irritating clothing, avoid chemicals in the form of hair dyes and makeup, give up the heeled shoes and note for yourself if it helps with the itching, pain and rashes. Above all it is our central nervous system that will enjoy the vacation from what is considered fashionable (read: uncomfortable). During Covid isolation so many of us have felt the wonderful respite of wearing sweat pants all day and night!

It is primarily men who determine women's fashion although as it is often said, women dress for other women, not for men! This could be more complex in the area of trans gender and gender fluid orientations; nonetheless, for all humans, comfort is paramount. We can all redefine what is fashionable and how we present ourselves to the world if we demand clothing that is healthy for our bodies and not made from toxic fabric. Taking care of our skin, the largest organ of the body, will reduce the amount of itching and rashes we experience as persons with fibromyalgia.

Hypnotherapy

"With hypnosis, we can help people modulate perceptions
in ways that are therapeutically helpful."
– David Spiegel

For those of us with chronic pain and other distressing physical and psychological conditions, the practice of changing our brains through relaxation and exercise regimes can be overwhelming. Mindfulness meditation is one way that we can work with our minds to improve our daily lives, but it takes time and discipline. What if there were a quicker way for therapists to teach us how to bring about relief from pain and chronic fatigue? The medical community is finding that hypnosis can be effective in that regard, although to this point there is little if any evidence-based research on the effects of hypnosis for those of us with fibromyalgia. Nonetheless, it sounds promising.[17]

In a June 12, 2017 *Globe and Mail* article, Adriana Barton writes of the "growing scientific support for hypnosis." She quotes Dr. David Spiegel's description of hypnosis as a "very powerful means of changing the way we use our minds to control perception and our bodies." Hypnosis is currently being used in Belgium, Canada and the US, among a host of other countries for a variety of conditions. Barton further discusses the work of Dr. Leora Kutner, "a pediatric psychologist who specializes in clinical hypnosis, a technique for leveraging the brain's healing abilities during a trance state."

---

[17] I suggest the work of Drs. Herbert and David Spiegel entitled *Trance and Treatment Clinical Uses of Hypnosis* for a better understanding.

Given the ways in which those of us with fibromyalgia, PTSD, and other chronic pain disorders rehash anxiety-ridden experiences that are stored in our memories, any non-invasive approach which could release us from the grip of the past offers hope. Most of us are hurting deep down in our psyches, and hypnotherapy may offer us a way to relinquish some of these painful memories.

On a lighter note, I once underwent hypnosis by a medical doctor dabbling in the practice, to work on my chocolate obsession. Five minutes after I left his office, I found myself in a candy store buying a chocolate bar. All that slow talking of his about candy only enhanced my desire for chocolate!

FMS and Cannabis

"I think people need to be educated to the
fact that [cannabis] is not a drug."
– Willie Nelson (*smile*)

There are many internet sites, articles and books that delve into the history of the Indian hemp plant cannabis. For the most part, the history of hemp is one of euphoria; other sources chronicle how the hemp plant itself was used in clothing and other products, rather than for medicinal purposes. In his book *Marijuana: The High and the Low,* Jerome Groopman writes that "Cannabis is one of the oldest psychotropic drugs in continuous use. Archaeologists have discovered it in digs in Asia that date to the Neolithic period around 4000 BCE." More recently, in 1839, a British doctor, William O'Shaughnessy wrote about its benefits and it became widespread for medical use, even prescribed to Queen Victoria for menstrual discomfort (cited in Groopman). Could this physician have imagined such a device as a gel pen filled with cannabis oil to apply locally? Or that there would be cannabis vaporizers, suppositories, oils, pills and other edibles, and even patches? Or, for that matter, the hundreds of slang terms that have evolved over the centuries of cannabis usage?

The medicinal effectiveness of cannabis has not been as carefully researched as that of prescription drugs. Much of the data on its medical uses are anecdotal; that's understandable since it is still illegal in most countries. Now that many American states have legalized its use, it is hoped that more participants will be willing to volunteer for larger studies without fear of repercussion. I am hopeful that Canada, where cannabis is legal, will lead the way in research.

To be realistic, the pharmaceutical industry is unlikely to pay for cannabis research so the problem of funding remains an issue, unless it can be shown to be profitable for the pharmaceutical companies. As a point of interest, the study conducted by Dr. Mark Ware and colleagues of McGill University in Montreal in 2016, write of the pharmaceutical development of cannabis patches for diabetic nerve pain and fibromyalgia. It is a small beginning for those of us with fibromyalgia and chronic pain, but a promising one.

Home growers of cannabis are of course somewhat leery about the legalization of cannabis in an increasing number of US jurisdictions, particularly if it is taken over by Big Pharma. Cannabis use is a social, political and medical issue that is very complex. Growing too much of a crop in one's yard is to be subject to criminality. And pharmaceutical companies may end up having complete control over some of countries where it is legal.

Before legalization, I was registered as a person who was legally allowed to use cannabis oil, taken orally for medical reasons. My fibromyalgia pain had increased tremendously since my hip replacement. Central sensitization had accelerated and flare-ups were more frequent with intense back pain from many degenerations of the lumbar spine. I had a choice: increase my dosage of Gabapentin or take an herb in the form of an oil. I chose the latter, despite still believing that most other herbs do not serve much purpose (although at least half of prescription drugs are plant-based, with added chemicals). I have concluded, after many years of reflecting and reading the science and hearing anecdotal testimonies, that cannabinoid usage is helpful for chronic pain, and what is more chronic than fibromyalgia? It is not a cure but a potential panacea.

So here I was, in the second month of experimenting with this wondrous herb called cannabis. It isn't easy trying to find the right mixture of THC to CBD, the two active ingredients, that agrees with a person's brain chemistry. Briefly stated, THC gives a person a "buzz" while CBD does not. CBD has been known to have medical benefits and can counteract THC lethargy. CBD is used for anxiety, pain, as an anti-inflammatory and antispasmodic. Finding the right combination is a slow process for each individual. Clearly, cannabis is not to be considered as "one size fits all." Even after two months of experimenting with dosage and time of day when I took it, I'm still learning about how much cannabis is right for anyone. But I was aided by my family physician and the very well-informed members of the National Access Cannabis Canada Clinic. The choices were mine and they involved reading, understanding and recording how each process was helping (or not).

A few years ago, my physiotherapist gave me a free sample of a topical cream of cannabis (PANAG Topical A -OTC). I began to use it for pain, and now regularly use CBD cream on various parts of my body and take CBD drops for pain.

Before legalization physicians could authorize (but not prescribe) the use of cannabis. However, some physicians would not even do that despite the patient's pain, especially the severe spasms common in multiple sclerosis. For those of us with fibromyalgia and other chronic pain, waiting for the legalities to be sorted out meant that we were expected to wait for treatment until the hysteria had subsided.

Clearly, in some circles there is still a stigma attached to cannabis use. In the words of the famous astronomer Carl Sagan: "The illegality of cannabis is outrageous, an impediment to full utilization of a drug which helps produce the serenity and insight, sensitivity and fellowship so desperately needed in this increasingly mad and dangerous world."

So-called cannabinophobia has resulted in a frenzy of political, medical, social and cultural chaos for generations in spite of the fact that this herb has been around for 38 million years. Prohibition against cannabis usage has resulted in billions of dollars wasted in policing its use, while hundreds of lives have been destroyed because of arrests, labelling recreational users as criminals.

It's time to lobby for world wide acceptance of an herb that can help with chronic pain and many other symptoms. We need to stop taking so many chemical prescriptions for pain whose long-term effects on our kidneys and liver are dangerous. Cannabis is a safe, effective, and non-addictive treatment for the symptoms of FMS.

In Canada the government legalized recreational cannabis in July 2018, the first of the G7 nations to do so. Currently in the US some states have legalized it for medical and recreational purposes. Many want to be open-minded about the topic, but it is far too often that their personal biases prevent reasonable discussions. While it is often said that religion, sex and politics are taboo subjects to be avoided in polite company, I believe cannabis should be added to that list as, like alcohol, it is a personal choice.

While I have many books on the benefits of cannabis, *The Pot Book: A Complete Guide to Cannabis* remains among my favourites, though it does not address FMS specifically. Searching through the hundreds of internet sites, published articles, and books on the subject is an ominous task, leaving the confused even more in a quandary. There is so little out there about the fibromyalgia pain, fatigue and malaise, (among a host of other symptoms) and using cannabis for treatment, that it is little wonder those of us with this syndrome wonder what should be done.

My view is that if alcohol, cigarettes and prescription medications are available as a panacea for stress, anxiety, depression and pain why not cannabis? If one can easily access cigarettes or imbibing alcohol for the social, recreational and personal pleasure of relaxation why isn't it the same for weed? Why is it legal to take a prescribed chemical such as valium or diazepam but not an herb, like cannabis?

In my own experience, most herbs, like the ones used in traditional Chinese medicine, had little effect on my FMS symptoms. The same was the case for Deb, another woman I interviewed, who tried dozens of alternative therapies for her FMS symptoms with no effect:

"Electro-dermal meridian assessments, Omega, acupressure points, NAET [a therapy which changes our energy field, and deprograms our brain], cleansing programs, homeopathy drops, therapeutic touch, accessing our energy fields, naturopaths, Juice Plus, many, many vitamins, hitting each knee with your opposite knee, acupuncture, having mercury removed from teeth. Oh, thousands and thousands of dollars. Some people take vacations. Mine is health."

When I first wrote about cannabinoids in 2009, I explained that I had never tried cannabis for FMS pain, nor for any other reason. I have never smoked a cigarette nor do I drink alcohol, the latter because it is too stimulating for me, not for any moral reason. I avoid caffeinated drinks for that same reason. I simply don't like the feeling of being out of control, and my central nervous system cannot tolerate stimulants. I have never taken a psychotropic drug, and other than Gabapentin and an occasional Tylenol, I suffer through unrelenting pain unmedicated. I am not a martyr, but until it was suggested I try cannabis, I believed there wasn't any hope for relief and the anecdotes I was reading about cannabis seemed encouraging. The hundreds of comments on my blog posts over the years have shown me just how many mood-altering drugs people are taking for their emotional wellbeing and to cope with the pain of fibromyalgia. Why not try the unknown, I thought? I was eager to try!

The risks of smoking tobacco are clear, and even printed on cigarette packages: especially the chance of developing lung cancer. The cigarettes that tobacco pickers made themselves burned the back of their throats when smoked. Over the years, many have told me and written about sensations of burning, coughing and wheezing they incur after smoking cannabis, particularly from unknown sources. Tobacco wasn't always regulated nor were the ingredients clearly stated on packages. If cannabis was regulated and ingredients stated before use, would buyers become more cautious about from whom they were buying? Would they switch to vaporized, oils, sprays, suppositories, even the new market of pills, or edible means of ingesting cannabis recreationally? Or is it the ritual of preparing, and sharing a smoke that is enjoyable?

Another factor to consider in the discussion about medical cannabis is the cost, which is often prohibitive when it comes in forms like CBD oil and patches (it takes more plant matter to produce these forms of cannabis, so the cost is higher). It's likely that those who are taking cannabis for pain are smoking it, as this is cheaper. Cost must always be considered as many people with fibromyalgia have had to stop working due to their pain and cannot afford an oil, vapour or patch.

In the last four years at one hospital in Denver it was said that there was a big increase in the number of young clients with nausea, abdominal cramps, vomiting due to cannabis. [18] The data has shown that the current level of THC in weed is six times more powerful than it was in the 1970s, and adolescent psychosis is an even more serious problem. It is speculated that using cannabis before the age of 25 is harmful to the brain. Yet, there is also anecdotal evidence that cannabis is helpful in some cases of children with such conditions as epilepsy and certainly in cancer-related situations.

It is an old idea that if cannabis is legalized worldwide, it will lead to addiction and the use of more dangerous drugs. A casual drinker of alcohol does not necessarily become an alcoholic so that issue is a moot point.

---

[18] Reported in *The Chronicle Herald*, November 16, 2016, A16

In states where cannabis is legal, like California, the drug is treated much like alcohol: you need to be 21 and over to buy it, and the state imposes a 15 percent sales tax on retail sales as well as additional taxes on growers. Legalizing cannabis could generate as much as $1 billion in tax revenue; cash-strapped jurisdictions could receive a huge boost from sales, so it's not surprising that more and more states are moving to decriminalize the recreational use of cannabis.

In the Appendix, you will find a short list of book titles that may be helpful as you navigate the complex world of cannabis as a pain reliever (and a political football!). I no longer take cannabis oil and it was only a brief foray into that world but I have wandered into a carefully regulated cannabis store and bought cannabis cream which is helpful when I have a flare -up on some part of my body. It is now a natural part of Canadian culture.

Telling Our Story: Writing About Fibromyalgia

"There is no greater agony than bearing an untold story inside you."
– Maya Angelou

I recently listened to a very interesting radio interview With Dr. Suzanne Koven, a Massachusetts General Hospital primary care doctor and writer in residence who writes, teaches and speaks about the healing power of story-writing. Her words have allowed me to ponder my own need to write about fibromyalgia, as well as what others have written in response to my blog posts on FMS. Though I no longer actively maintain my blog, for many years, it was a shared community for those of us with fibromyalgia. Writing about our shared condition has also allowed me to reflect upon the process of accepting that I have a lifelong challenge ahead of me.

I frequently review sites about fibromyalgia and while many come and go, I wonder at my own need to continue, year after year, to write about the many issues that plague those of us living with this invisible dis-ease. Are we all alike in this daily struggle? Or is there one symptom that hounds us more than others? For me it is undoubtedly pain, though anxiety and depression can actually be more debilitating and eventually turn into pain and fatigue. In my view, FMS is a mental health issue first and foremost, as it involves a great deal of ruminating about the past and looking anxiously toward the future.

Among the many symptoms of FMS I experience, my lack of stamina distresses me greatly since I was once a high-energy person. The past is always there waiting, reminding me of what I used to be able to do. Life can send us reeling, dealing us blows we struggle to recover from, presenting us with sometimes unreliable memories. Yet, it is in telling the story of my life in writing that I can now see a pattern, a series of events that overwhelmed my nervous system's ability to deal with life challenges. I reclaim some of this loss through therapeutic writing.

As a mindful writer I work to get difficult thoughts out of my head and then out of my body. I know enough about neuroplasticity to realize that who I am is malleable and can be changed. The past and the future are not the present; they are created in the brain. While the past impacts my present, I must "re-engage the healthy self," in the words of Dr. Koven. I engage this self in the therapeutic act of writing and sharing my story.

Judgement and problem-solving about our emotions are difficult. It often shows how little we know about ourselves. In *The Science of Storytelling* by Will Storr and *Mindwise* by Nicholas Epley, it is underscored that we can't change our behaviour without understanding the source, nor can we know ourselves without delving into the root cause of how we became the way we are. Writing is one way we come to know ourselves better.

When I was actively writing blog posts, I enjoyed long comments from readers as it reiterated my view that there is a healing power in storytelling. I decided to try my hand at offline writing about personal issues after reading an article that referenced the work of Dr. Richard Davidson, founder of the Center for Healthy Minds at the University of Wisconsin-Madison, and a specialist in the neuroscience of emotion. Dr. Davidson presented us with the interesting option of "spending as little as 30 minutes per day training our minds to do something different [than focusing on our usual anxieties]"[19] which can result in changing the brain. Writing seemed to fit that bill.

I began to write short stories about my life, exploring reasons why I am the way I am: an anxious person with a tendency to overreact to any kind of stimulation, setting off a cascade of pain and fatigue flare-ups. Writing in short bursts of two or three pages about events in my life, for example, about my first day of school, would often bring about unhappy memories, though intended as a therapeutic exercise.

---

[19] *Mindful* magazine, August 2014, 52.

I shared this sad story with two friends, who each had a had different reaction to it. One friend suggested it was a good practice to write down bad memories, print them, then tear them up and discard them forever. The other friend reminded me about how writing could reactivate the amygdala and cause me to relive a bad experience; in short, they thought writing about past trauma was not a good idea.

Several research studies have suggested that writing about trauma helps us to make meaning of what happened to us, which can help us with processing the trauma and moving on.[20] It is important, though, for those of us with fibromyalgia and PTSD to listen to our own bodies for distress cues if what we are writing is causing us to reactivate our symptoms.

Memory can be a rich source of both pleasure and pain as we relive our past. We would be wise to recall the words of the Buddha in this regard: "The secret of health for both mind and body is not to mourn for the past, worry about the future, or anticipate troubles, but to live in the present moment wisely and earnestly." There are strategies for improving memory focus. A course from the Harvard Health Harvard Medical School is a wonderful program to help with cognitive issues. https://www.health.harvard.edu/topics/memory

---

[20] See for example, Park, C.L., Blumberg, C.J. Disclosing Trauma Through Writing: Testing the Meaning-Making Hypothesis. *Cognitive Therapy and Research* **26**, 597–616 (2002). https://doi.org/10.1023/A:1020353109229

Touch-based Therapies Revisited

"Touch seems to be as essential as sunlight."
– Diane Ackerman

I have discussed manual therapy in earlier sections of this book but would like to revisit the topic in a more organized way as I recognize how many kinds of touch-based therapy exist.

For those of us with FMS, manual therapy can offer varying degrees of relief for our debilitating symptoms. Not only is there often a sense of relief in experiencing the healing touch of a professional as the muscles and the nervous system both relax, but the person being touched often feels a sense of awareness of the connection of the body and mind, along with a deep sense of well being. These positive sensations also remind us that we do remember what it feels like to feel good!

Let me list a few professionals whom I have consulted with and present my own analysis of their effectiveness for me personally:

Massage therapy

In Canada we have very strict guidelines for who can become a Registered Massage Therapist. Their educational system consists of a two-year program and they must pass difficult standardized exams before they can qualify to practice as RMTs. Their knowledge of anatomy and physiology is extensive. Many of their clients suffer from chronic pain, among them people with fibromyalgia. The more experienced ones are highly regarded as their knowledge is invaluable.

I have found massage helpful, although its effects were not long-lasting. Sometimes though, I found that too much was "stirred up" after a massage treatment and I would have after-effects. Gentle soothing strokes like those used in Russian massage, which is only 30 minutes in duration, do help; this style of massage has been found to be evidence-based, which is unusual for massage practices.

The downside of massage therapy is the cost. Many, especially those who are no longer able to work or who only work part-time, cannot afford the luxury of massages. Even bartering with someone close to you can be problematic as trying to massage someone can cause a flare-up of hand, neck or back pain. In lieu of this, I suggest gentle self-massage with perhaps a feather on legs or arms as a way of making contact with the nervous system; it can be relaxing.

More and more evidence of gentle massage is shown to have beneficial effects for the elderly in long-term care settings. In the olden days of back rubs in hospitals, patients looked forward to that three-times-a-day practice from the nurses' soothing hands.

While I have had many forms of massage, I do enjoy reflexology, where pressure is applied to specific points on the feet, ears, and/or hands, because it is so gentle, although it is generally not considered a genuine massage practice in and of itself.

Chiropractic adjustments

I have generally found these to be helpful as my body often feels out of alignment; a short 15-to-20-minute adjustment sometimes helps the joints. However, I am sometimes sore for a day or two afterwards, even if it does not hurt at the time. I am never sure if a flare-up is caused by this therapy.

As with massage therapy, the cost of chiropractic treatments may be prohibitive for those without medical insurance, and if one does not have joint issues, mild exercise may be the way to go rather than more dramatic chiropractic adjustments.

Both chiropractors and osteopaths lay claim to being able to adjust the spinal column; however, only chiropractic professionals have graduated from a school which is largely evidence-based. Chiropractors are experts in anatomy and physiology and spend four years studying to become a Doctor of Chiropractic (DC). They can not only order x-rays but can take them if their clinic has the facilities.

Chiropractors base their practice on the belief that bones are out of place, that the spine is out of alignment, though many mainstream medical practitioners dispute the existence of "subluxations"[21] (or "partial abnormal separation[s] of the articular surfaces of a joint") which form the basis for chiropractic practice.

The jury is out as to whether chiropractic manual therapy is a true science or not. Even if it generates a placebo effect, my view is, if it seems to release pain, keep up with it! If it doesn't, then search for other forms of touch that can provide relief, even if only temporary. This form of treatment should never hurt. For me a chiropractic appointment is very helpful and my favourite form of relief from physical pain.

Osteopathy

What is an osteopath? In the US, it is a medical doctor who then takes training as a doctor of osteopathy but functions as a regular general practitioner. In Canada and some parts of Europe, it is a rather different story. A DO is a diploma-trained osteopath, not a medical doctor with a degree. These practitioners cannot be called "doctor" from their study of osteopathy, and upon graduation they receive a diploma rather than a university degree.

The founder of osteopathy was a man by the name of Andrew Still who was disillusioned by his studies in allopathic (conventional) medicine and did not finish medical school. Instead, he began a school of his own in the US in the 1800s where students extensively studied bones. In that respect his work was evidence-based for the times as he intensively studied the bone structures of cadavers and became expert in their functions.

Osteopathy, as it became known, is a type of alternative medicine in which manual treatments are given to attempt to relieve muscle and skeletal problems in preference to pharmaceuticals. It can be gentle and soothing, and experienced osteopaths use their hands to guide treatment.

---

[21] https://www.spine-health.com

Still's student William Garner Sutherland originated the idea of applying osteopathy to the cranial field. He believed that cranial bone mobility would affect cerebral spinal fluid pressure. Later scientific evidence would repudiate this observation, though the practice of craniosacral therapy has persisted among some osteopaths and massage therapists.

Many practitioners believe that by releasing the bones of the cranium the cerebral spinal fluid is regulated and pain can be released. There are many who believe that by releasing these bones even fibromyalgia may be helped. None of these assumptions have been proven to be totally true. Research has shown a therapist cannot move the bones of the skull enough, if at all, to affect the circulation of the spinal cord.

Rather than go into too much detail on the history of osteopathy, it is sufficient to say that, like massage therapists or anyone who practices any kind of manual therapy, an intuitive understanding of the muscles and bones evolves over a long time. On the downside, osteopathy is not an evidence-based practice and is expensive for the client as it is often not paid for by insurance companies.

Interestingly, in Canada it is often massage therapists who want the extra perceived prestige of a diploma in osteopathy after their names who enrol in this kind of training. However, in the long run I believe it is their initial training in massage and the years of experience they have accrued which often guides their practice.

I have had osteopathic manual therapy from an experienced practitioner, and can attest to a degree of effectiveness for a short period of time, but not for a long-standing condition like fibromyalgia. It is a syndrome that requires more than manual therapy to treat. However, those of us who enjoy the stroking, rubbing, touching, and massaging of our aching bodies, the relaxation aspect of osteopathy can be pleasant, and if one can afford it, and way to train the nervous system to relax and the muscles to move. My personal preference is chiropractic adjustments.

Physiotherapy (Physical Therapy)

Here we find one of the respected, evidence-based professions that almost always uses manual therapies to treat the body. Some PTs, of course, use electrodes, the machines that take the place of hands and allow the physiotherapist to treat more than one client at a time. I am critical of this practice, as it does not lead to the soothing experience that we as FMS sufferers require to calm our nervous systems.

Insurance companies will fund physiotherapy claims if one is fortunate to have access to insurance. In publicly-funded hospitals, these are the professionals who are employed as manual therapists and there are many in private practice. Physiotherapy schools are situated in universities where the professors are expected to do research that is scientific in nature. Physiotherapy is not considered to be an "alternative medicine" approach, but mainstream. I will mention a few of the approaches of the more recent forms of physiotherapy:

A **simple contact** approach, developed by Barrett Dorko, utilizes the body's own subconscious movement, called *ideomotor movement*. I would encourage the reader to explore this concept as I have found it to be most helpful in the past. Ideomotion is a non-voluntary physical movement prompted by mental activity. An example of this is the pain in my left hip; the hip wants to move in certain ways but is prevented from moving by my brain registering pain. This pain has been released through the gentle and slow movement of my leg by the physiotherapist. With this gentle, relaxing approach, I can "be in the moment" without worrying about the possibility of pain.

Gentle skin stretching, called **dermoneuromodulation** (DNM) was developed by physiotherapist Diane Jacobs as a tissue glide in directions the body likes. I have had the privilege of having treatments by Ms. Jacobs while she was living in Vancouver. These are words taken from her website: "Dermoneuromodulating, or -tion, is a structured, interactive approach to manual therapy that considers the nervous system of the patient from skin cell to sense of self. Techniques are slow, light, kind, intelligent, responsive and effective." Her blogs and websites are nothing less than amazing, and her approach is one to which I ascribe.

Somatic exercises were developed by Thomas Hanna to help contract the reflexive muscles so that one can actively own the muscle again, overriding the pain reflex. Such treatments include yoga, Pilates and the Feldenkrais technique, and there are many therapists who employ these methods which come under the umbrella of massage or physiotherapy.

Craniofacial work*: A more recent approach is that of Harry J.M. von Piekartz (author of *Craniofacial Pain: Neuromusculoskeletal Assessment, Treatment and Management)* which is similar to the craniosacral perspective of osteopaths, some chiropractors, and massage therapists. This work is considered by many to be evidence-based and grounded in pain science research for those suffering from craniofacial challenges. The work of Von Piekartz has become very popular among many physiotherapists worldwide, but not as much in Canada, where I live. His technique seems to be about changing sensory input to the brain; all nerves pass from the skull into lower regions of the body. This style of craniosacral massage is gentle and not at all painful. I have enjoyed it.

All the manual therapies I have discussed here are helpful for those suffering from FMS, as long as they are done gently, and a person can afford them. Because touch is so important to calming our nervous system, all of these techniques feel good. Especially for those with fibromyalgia, touching is relaxing, and provides the brain with proof that there is pleasure in life.

We fibromyalgia people are what our ancestors once called "highly strung." We need to work with, not against the nervous system and manual therapists can help if they are up to date about the brain research and their views are evidence-based. In the meantime, a simple back or foot rub from a loving person might suffice.

Before beginning a course of manual therapy treatment, please consider the following: while stretching and various exercises are always advocated by physiotherapists, the stretches must be very gentle or a severe flare-up might ensue. It has happened to me on many occasions. Filled with enthusiasm and desire for a new regime of exercise I have failed to heed my own warning. So go slow, be gentle and do not overdo it.

Daily Life with Chronic Pain

"In three words I can sum up everything I've
learned about life: it goes on."
– Robert Frost

I have frequently cited chronic pain self-management writer Bronnie Lennox Thompson who blogs at https://healthskills.wordpress.com. She has become my guru for updates on research regarding pain. I take hope because of her personal struggles with living with acceptance in lieu of catastrophizing.

Daily pain is exhausting, depletes our energy, and leaves us with a sense of hopelessness. Each new symptom (and there are many) can be like taking one step forward and two backward. How do we continue? As Bronnie says in her October 18, 2015 blog: "After all, life doesn't stop just because pain is a daily companion." The same could be said of the other myriad of symptoms those of us with fibromyalgia experience.

Chronic pain is one of the leading reasons for doctor's visits, workday losses, and prescriptions for pharmaceuticals. Health care professionals are trying many strategies to ease the suffering of millions of us with a compromised quality of life. Among these professionals is the American law professor Toni Bernhard, who documents her journey through the maze of adapting to and living fully with chronic illness. One of her books is a practical and honest account of the ways in which a person living with chronic illness can turn their lives around. *How to Live Well with Chronic Pain and Illness* is invaluable. Mindfulness meditation is integral to Bernhard's work (see my earlier discussion of mindfulness meditation).

It would seem that the advice of most chronic pain experts is very similar: exercise moderately when able, meditate, learn to say "no," avoid being around friends and family who do not support you, pace your activities, practice self compassion and above all learn to live, rather than defining yourself as your pain. Living in the past or looking into the future is counterproductive. Being in the moment is the only way to live life fully.

It has taken me a long time to stop thinking like an invalid, rather than to acknowledge that I will live with pain but it will not define me. I will continue to do things I enjoy, with limitations, rather than waiting for the pain and fatigue to overtake me. But oftentimes I give in to hopelessness, particularly when my energy is depleted. It is difficult to accept that monitoring myself is the "new normal."

Bronnie Thompson writes: "We all know that having pain can act as a disincentive to doing things. What's less clear is how, when a person is in chronic pain, life can continue" (October 18, 2015). She goes on to say how complicated it is to work around what is considered to be "normal" within daily living. Life never proceeds along a linear straight path without daily fluctuations. What is normal on a snowy, blustery, isolating day differs from what we do on a lovely, sunny autumn day when getting around outside is less problematic. Some things (like Covid-related restrictions) are beyond our control while others are of our own doing.

Trying to organize a dinner party for a dozen family friends at Thanksgiving is a major undertaking. But taking a drive in the countryside to leisurely appreciate the beauty of the day can be soothing. Yet, both are what we might enjoy and having to exclude the one that would cause stress and anxiety might produce feelings of guilt and sadness. But serving and preparing a dinner for guests can also result in catastrophic thinking as one usually tries to be the perfect host.

In the past I would have exhausted myself trying to manage the entire affair. It takes a great deal of courage to be present at an occasion and not organize and take care of others. It takes old age to recognize that I can do both. Go for a ride to see the colours; go to a Thanksgiving dinner that someone else prepared and sit back, watching others, being thankful I can be there and not feeling overwhelmed with anxiety about how I should take charge.

After my month-long participation at the pain clinic, I began to realize that those of us with chronic pain fit a similar profile. Many of us are prone to catastrophizing about our symptoms, often give in to depression following a bout of anxiety over some new experience of pain, and generally cannot remember that life varies often from hour to hour, certainly day to day. That there are challenges for us there is little doubt, but the term *chronic* implies that these challenges are permanent, without any joy left to look forward to. Little wonder we give in to a sense of despair.

How many of us have fearful thoughts about the future? I do often. Believing I cannot ever again undertake a task that gives me joy is a challenge I face daily. We often have to compromise on our activities, but sometimes the brilliant ways in which we are able to modify our accomplishments can be very satisfying. I can no longer be the runner I once was, nor can I walk very far anymore without pain, but I can ride my recumbent bike with painless ease.

I have been reading how Buddhism defines destructive emotions as passion, aggression, and ignorance. I can relate this concept to fibromyalgia. Unless we become the expert of our own lives, we will continue to suffer from *ignorance* about this syndrome. Ignorance is at the root of our inability to see the truth about our relationship to our over-stimulated central nervous system. If we continue to treat fibromyalgia with *aggression* rather than with kindness, then we only exacerbate the symptoms. Without self-compassion we will continue to treat ourselves in ways that cause more suffering. Then there is *passion* which is the desire for a different life than what we have, a common wish for those with FMS.

I am not a Buddhist nor an expert on Buddhist philosophy, but one of the basic concepts is that of universal suffering. This suffering can be translated into anxiety or stress, the pains of growing old, and illness, all of which are endemic to fibromyalgia. We all suffer; it is part of the human condition. However, there is also joy. So, on a grey November day when the leaves have almost all fallen from the trees and we wait for the first snow in my part of the world, I have to practice what I preach. Stop and enjoy some of the beauty still left from the autumn colours.

On Being Our Own Physician

"He's the best physician that knows the
worthlessness of most medicines."
– Benjamin Franklin

I was fortunate for many decades to have a physician who was sympathetic to my condition, highly intelligent and comforting, and did not suggest unnecessary tests. I would be the last to engage in doctor-bashing. Still, I am aware of the runaround that many people with chronic pain experience as they "doctor shop."

Physicians do not want their patients to suffer. However, often they are stymied by the host of symptoms presented to them which cannot be explained. For that reason, many people are burdened with a deluge of medical tests without receiving any concrete explanation about their condition.

When patients present themselves to their health care providers with chronic pain and a myriad of other invisible symptoms, their desire is for relief, and more importantly, a cure. It is reasonable at first to rule out life-threatening conditions with testing, but with fibromyalgia these tests can go on and on for several years or longer.

I was 25 and recovering from a difficult delivery via C-section when I had my first attack of fibromyalgia. I could barely walk. I was diagnosed with gout! I was a small person and did not have any of the usual characteristics of the gout patient, but this misdiagnosis kept me from understanding the side effects of the many medications I began taking. For many years, various tests kept me wondering anxiously what each one would reveal (in the end, nothing was revealed!) The pain continued and has to this day.

I have recently seen a website where a physician who herself has fibromyalgia suggests that a particular product has become the treatment of choice for both herself and her patients with whom she has had great success. I have read many such claims over the years and I find them disheartening. There is no evidence-based medical treatment that has been shown to cure fibromyalgia. As for supplements, there are no long-term studies that can say with a fair degree of certainty that people with fibromyalgia are insufficient in magnesium, potassium, phosphorus, or any other kind of vitamin or mineral deficiency.

It seems likely that after years of pain and the many other symptoms of this syndrome, that changes can eventually occur within the body which may have a deleterious effect on the hormonal and endocrine system, (and perhaps, as in my case, the cardiovascular system). But to date, none of this can be proven. Fibromyalgia remains an elusive condition of primarily pain, fatigue and a host of other symptoms that in the short-term are non-life threatening. I can only repeat what I have been proselytizing for many years: **pain is in the brain**. The pattern of more and more tests to make this invisible dis-ease fit a disease paradigm is exhausting, expensive and unnecessary.

Does this leave us without hope? Absolutely not. While it is challenging, brain research of the last two decades has shown the ability of the brain to change. But more tests, more misdiagnoses, useless medications, and constant physician visits are not the answer. Interventions that are intended to promote self-management are the way that we should move forward as we become the experts of our own lives. But then I am repeating myself. It is a struggle managing pain and fatigue, but any elixir that is said to cure fibromyalgia is not addressing the hyper-sensitive, hyper-aroused nervous system of those of us who are seeking a cure.

How can we be our own physicians, or case managers, when we suffer from chronic pain? A popular approach to pain management is a form of therapy called "acceptance and commitment (ACT)," developed in the 1980s by psychologist Steven Hayes and his colleagues (see Appendix for ACT resources.) Primarily this means an acceptance that one does have pain that frequently recurs, yet we can also go on to engage in those things in life that give us pleasure. In short, it is a commitment to pleasurable activities by not engaging in negative thoughts about the pain, what caused it, and all memories of the past experiences of this pain. This kind of therapy, in my view, can be as effective as mindfulness. It is possible to change the brain through discipline and consistent letting go of the thoughts that reinforce the feelings associated with the pain. Accepting pain does not deny its existence or mean that we are giving in to it. By accepting pain, we do not waste precious energy on struggling against it, nor do we allow it to become the centre of our lives.

When pain appears, I tell it I haven't the time to think about it right now. I tell the pain, "I will make an appointment with you later on, but for now I am letting you go from my thoughts." I wish I could say that I am always successful with this strategy; of course, it doesn't mean the pain has disappeared. Rather, it helps me to live life as fully as I can by accepting my dis-abilities rather than giving in to hopelessness. It is giving my neurons a message to take to the brain that is less anxiety- provoking.

On Overdoing it

"If there is no struggle, there is no progress."
– Frederick Douglass

There is a tendency among those of us with chronic pain to be extremely watchful on days when we are in pain or are very fatigued. We take it easy on those days and begin to wonder if we will ever be feeling well again. But then, on those days when we are feeling well, our tendency is to be optimistic, think we are cured, and immediately do more than we should. We then pay for our burst of energy with a big flare-up. It is usually one step forward, one step backward. Sound familiar?

How do we make sense of feeling great one day and lousy the next? What is it about us that cannot seem to predict what will bring on a flare-up if we overdo it on a good day? I think the latter situation occurs when our brain remembers life before FMS and becomes excited. We are feeling well and want more of that feeling; we deceive ourselves that we can go beyond the limits of yesterday when we did not feel so great. It is a series of ups and downs. We refuse to listen to warnings that one cannot be almost bedridden one day and up for a hike the next. Our brains deceive us; we become weary of thinking of ourselves as "pain people." We crave normality. We want to go to that family gathering that inevitably overstimulates us, just as we have wanted to go back to "normal" social interaction during Covid-19. We want to take an hour-long walk instead of a 15 minute one because the day is so nice, filled with sunshine. The sky is the limit on what we can do on that magical day. Then the sky falls down and we are once again down and out the next day or the day after that. Our brains have not yet recognized that if we continually fail at some tasks, repeating them will mean we get the same results!

How can we learn to pace ourselves? It may help to chart our energy expenditures each day to make ourselves aware of how we are spending this precious and limited resource. The Parkwood Institute in London, Ontario, a leader in helping people recover from mild traumatic brain injury, developed a system called Pacing Points, where each activity of daily life is assigned a point value based on how much energy is required to complete it. A good energy budget may be around 12 to 15 points per day, which we get to choose how we will spend. We also get to assign point values to activities based on how depleted we feel when we do them. For example, a phone call with an understanding friend may be soothing to our nervous system and only account for 0.5 points, while a stressful interaction with our boss or watching an upsetting newscast may cost us 5 points.[22] We need to limit our exposure to stressful encounters by noticing how much energy they cost us.

Cognitive therapy, which teaches us to notice our own habitual patterns and helps us to change them is an evidence-based program that can help with the tendency to overdo! In the meantime, "Keep calm and carry on" as the old WW2 saying goes. Calm is a balm for fibromyalgia.

---

[22] To watch a short video about the Parkwood Institute's Pacing Points program, visit https://www.sjhc.london.on.ca/regional-acquired-brain-injury-program/patients/activity-and-exercise

"Alternative Therapies"

"People still insist on things like holistic healing and
things that have no real basis in evidence because
they want it to be true—it's as simple as that."
– Stephen Fry

In the past several decades, there has been a proliferation of alternative and complementary medicines which claim to be able to treat the symptoms of fibromyalgia. This is not surprising, given that people in chronic pain become frustrated with living with their condition and want immediate help and cure; many are desperate enough to try anything. Energy healing, acupuncture, so-called natural herbs and concoctions will not cure FMS, as we have seen that it is a condition that is bio-psycho-social in nature. The treatment for fibro lies within us. We are the expert of our own lives.

It is important for us to explore the most up-to-date brain research and its impact on the biological and psychological aspects of pain, along with the symptoms that develop from years of living with chronicity. It is researchers such as David Butler, Lorimer Mosley and Diane Jacobs who can keep us up to date about the new science-based evidence regarding the brain.

We often hear of "experts" who postulate that those with FMS have less or more of this or that in our endocrine or hormonal systems. A study here and there suggests we have such-and-such wrong with our bodies that makes us different from the "norm" and suddenly a cause is discovered. There is little doubt that after a long episode of this syndrome, various systems in the body become debilitated, but one study that explores an organ or certain capacities or inabilities of fibromyalgia subjects is not scientific evidence! Repeated long term, double blind, peer reviewed studies of the biology of fibromyalgia have yet to be done. We are so quick to find symptoms rather than explore cause.

Numerous claims are made by those who practice or have beliefs in pseudoscience (also called "woo-woo"); they endorse various concoctions, herbs, homeopathic solutions (sugar pills) and other types of unproven remedies or "therapies" that will cure fibromyalgia. I am biased towards that which has been tested scientifically, in spite of the fact that there can be mistakes made within the realm of science. There are two choices: scientific medicine which is evidence- based or complementary/alternative medicine which has not been validated with rigour. But I have not always been so discerning.

In the past I have spent hundreds of dollars on herbs, homeopathy, magnetic therapy…the list is endless. It is a very expensive path to follow. I believe I have tried them all and with no positive results, except perhaps temporarily due to the placebo effect. I speak from experience. Yet, I also know that conventional medicine also does not have an answer for those of us with fibromyalgia, except through quieting our untamed nervous systems as shown from the brain research evidence. Some of us do somewhat better with some kinds of medication that help with pain, but they are not a cure. Drugs will not cure fibromyalgia and the search for ones that will is futile.

Over the years I have been a fan of James Randi and his exposition of all that is pseudo-science. I refer the readers to the James Randi Educational Foundation or www.randi.org.

While in his eighties, Randi was relentless in his desire to continue to uncover the ways in which those who espouse magic cures or treatments dupe the public. Homeopathy, in particular, has been exposed as one of the primary culprits. We would do well to save our money and become the expert of our own lives, utilizing strategies that have been shown to change the brain, that will lead us down pathways that are more productive and certainly less expensive. Not easy when what we wish for is an easy fix from that homeopathic bottle of water!

I am also a big fan of scientist Neil de Grasse Tyson: no woo-woo from him or Randi, just the scientific facts! In the words of David Suzuki, "Science is the most powerful way of knowing."

And now to "energy medicine." Given that modern medicine has been unable to find either a cause or cure for fibromyalgia, it is little wonder that many have turned to an alternate way of viewing and discussing the body in order to deal with the many daily issues facing them. "Energy medicine" is significant in that it has changed the discourse about the body and is the approach that is popular with those who are not mainstream health care practitioners, although, in fact, even some conventional practitioners embrace the paradigm, which continues to amaze me.

Generally based upon therapies that evolved from Eastern philosophies, this belief system involves a "healer," body/mind techniques, and a strong emphasis on self-healing. Advocates believe that it is a cure for many ailments, among them fibromyalgia, chronic fatigue, and environmental illness.

From discussions about meridians, emotional freedom techniques, qi gong, therapeutic touch (TT), reiki, theta healing (where the healer evokes a higher power then commands a specific healing), pranic healing (another form of non-touch energy healing, like TT), power healing, (mantra chanting to shake energy loose) acupuncture, and even auras and chakras, I have been left with more questions than answers as the language of energy medicine is both perplexing and mystical. How do you we know whether meridians, auras or chakras actually exist? If they do exist, why can't they be seen? We can see nerves within the nervous system and actually measure brain activity, but we can't find meridians (apparently there are 14 of these pathways in the body) which are said to carry energy into and out of the body. Where exactly are the chakras which are believed to be the concentrated center of energy in the body? If the aura is thought to be a shell that emanates from the body and intersects with energy in the body, why can't we find it?

Other important questions: where is the qi (chi or ch'i) which is not detectable by empirical science but integral to all these practices? Is it similar to the soul which also cannot be seen, but many believe in? Do we have to have blind faith to believe that qi exists? How does tapping on the presumed meridians of certain body parts (as in emotional freedom techniques) release negative emotions by unblocking qi, which is supposedly an energy that permeates everything and flows along the meridians? I have done qi gong for the exercise component which, like tai chi, is useful for movement purposes. I've also tried EFT and jin shin, which I loved—I like all forms of gentle touch which serve to quiet my nervous system— but I never believed I was tapping into meridians nor moving electrical currents through these meridians.

The biggest question of all is why the language of the nervous system, nerve function and brain activity (about which a great deal of empirical evidence has been known for decades) has become permeated by the language of energy medicine, which does not have a correlation with organs and nerves? It is interesting to me to find the conversion of scientifically-trained physicians, nurses, pharmacists and physiotherapists who have embraced energy medicine in rather great numbers.

Acupuncture has pinpointed (no pun intended!) 500 specific points in which sticking needles into body parts can open up blocked qi. Is there some possible explanation about why many patients experience relief from chronic pain with acupuncture? Perhaps this is due to the placebo effect, or acupuncture could be said to block the transmission of pain from various areas in the body to the central nervous system. Equally as possible, it is likely that sticking needles into, or pressing on, certain points on the body affects the nervous system and stimulates endorphins and releases serotonin, bringing relief. We simply do not know specifically how acupuncture helps in pain control in some people.

Though I have not personally found long-lasting relief through alternative/ complementary medicine, I do respect the good intent of those in the alternate paradigm to bring about an awareness of the body/ mind connection with fibromyalgia. There is little doubt that the nervous system needs an approach that can tame the turmoil that plagues our everyday existence. But believing that tapping myself on various parts of the body (EMT) is going to release stuck energy in the meridians fails to convince me of its efficacy. Strengthening exercises and practicing relaxing mindfulness meditation on a daily basis helps calm the nervous system and is much cheaper and more effective (in my experience) for fibromyalgia than going to expensive practitioners who purport to cure fibromyalgia.

Finding Your Own Pace

"If you can anchor yourself to a ship of tranquility, you
won't be tossed about by the waves of stimulation."
– Ted Zeff

I recently asked my spouse what lessons he had learned from his father. His reply was how to pace himself, to be cautious and not overly frenetic. His father lived to be 90, was a factory worker and a musician, and helped raise five children. He was a calm man, did not complain about aches or pains, was easygoing and like his son, my partner of many years, a relaxed man. He was like this in spite of the stimulation of having five children and two jobs. It was a pleasure to be around him. He moved about slowly, pacing himself. Neither he nor his son have, nor had fibromyalgia. That goes without saying.

By contrast, my father, even in his nineties, lived a life of intense anxiety, fear, stress, and anger; he complained about his body's aches and pains his whole life. He caused stress and agitation to all around him with his emotional outbursts. Everything he did was done quickly and often carelessly. He taught me to be fearful and to rush through life, never letting up. He would never know what it means to pace oneself. He said he could not sleep at night if he knew something had to be done; his example was changing a malfunctioning electric socket in a wall! In fact, he complained that he couldn't sleep at night anyway. Somewhat miraculously, he lived to be 92, always fearful and never slowing down.

A Buddhist therapist told me of a religious leader who once said that when we are born, it is as though we are presented with a smorgasbord of personality characteristics to choose from: some of us will choose joy, fearlessness, and optimism, while others will choose anxiety, depression, fear, and anger to be our main life traits. Many of us choose a mix of traits while others choose extremes. Needless to say, we usually take on these personality characteristics based upon our parents' ways of being in the world. If we see a great deal of anger in one parent, we may choose fear as the safety measure to guide us through life. If we feel the need to rush about helping others (whether they need it or not), rushing through our days, wanting everything done yesterday, how can we take care of ourselves?

But how can we pace ourselves in the activities of daily living when we are frenetically sensitive to all stimuli that urge us toward constant activity? We buzz around from one chore to another that needs not be done immediately and burn ourselves out by early afternoon. Learning to organize a manageable routine, and planning from one activity to the next, requires discipline. In his book *The Highly Sensitive Person's Guide*, Ted Zeff writes, "Perhaps when you are in an overstimulating situation a good question to ask yourself would be how you can feel more in control of circumstances rather than being a victim of stimuli?" (p.14)

Zeff's book is one I recommend for highly sensitive persons. The strategies for living life in the slow lane are key for those of us suffering from the angst of daily pain and fatigue which often inhibits our ability to live life as we formerly did.

Aging with Fibromyalgia

"To be seventy years young is sometimes far more
cheerful and hopeful than to be forty years old."
– Oliver Wendell Holmes

As we age, each new year brings hope of change in a positive direction. Less pain, less fatigue, and better-quality sleep are the things I wish for. My new year's resolutions: try not to overdo it like I always do on days when a flare-up has subsided; daily gentle exercises if only for a few minutes off and on each day; maybe take a music appreciation class. I would also like to practice meditation more regularly; try new creative things but only gradually, not like I did with the quilting: I had never quilted before and by hand I had sewed four quilts since Easter, without a sewing machine, giving myself carpal tunnel syndrome!

Some say that as one ages the nervous system of the person with fibro subsides and there are fewer and fewer flare-ups. The logic behind this idea seems to be that as our children grow up and leave home and our lives become more controlled and pleasant, we have less to be anxious about, and our pain should subside. I talk about that research in my first book. I want to go on record as saying that for me this has not been the case. My worries have not abated with the passing years: I spent much time caring for my elderly parents, and worrying about my adult children and family relationships, and the state of the world generally.

So, I would say that as we age fibromyalgia does not become easier. Living as I do in a cold climate there is always the weather to contend with as arthritis sets in to make the pain even less tolerable during the winter months.

I often wonder if the brain fog is just part of the aging process and not necessarily from fibromyalgia. The pain I experience upon exercise could also be from growing older.

In spite of this gloomy perspective, I do have hope for a better year as I am always looking for the silver lining and I know it is out there in the hands of the neuroscientists who are finding ways of changing the brain and especially working with chronic pain. Don't miss those PBS documentaries on pain and the brain and keep looking for positive and optimistic messages they convey for those of us who suffer with this demon, no matter what our ages happen to be! It **is** easier to change the brain of younger people but it is **never** too late to teach an old dog new tricks. It is just slower.

Healing Ourselves

"What I am looking for is not out there; it is in me."
– Helen Keller

To sum up what I've written about elsewhere in the book, my suggestions for the best ways to treat fibromyalgia are:

1) Remapping the brain
2) Controlling the excess arousal of the nervous system
3) Unlearning what we have believed to be either a biological/viral/bacterial cause of fibromyalgia
4) Stopping talk therapy after awhile because that only brings up the same negative stories we have told ourselves over and over and continues to reactivate our nervous stem
5) Stopping the search for a "cure" with medications.

Instead, I recommend the following:

1) Mindfully living moment to moment by attending to the stress, anxiety and pain in our lives through being aware of the actual bodily responses to them, that is, where in the body do we feel the pain or stress at this moment? As Schwartz and Begley have written in "The Mind and the Brain: Neuroplasticity and the Power of Mental Force": "The most noteworthy result of mindfulness, which requires directed willful effort, is the ability it affords those practicing it to observe their sensations and thoughts with the calm clarity of an external witness..." (p.11)

2) Diaphragmatic breathing,
3) Movement, such as gentle yoga, tai chi, qi gong, or if those are too strenuous, then walking for short periods frequently every day. Feeling too lousy for even a short walk? Stop now and shake your body, move your arms, shrug your shoulders: your body needs it. Do this often during the day.

Meditation for a few minutes each day may be helpful but without actual movement while being aware of feelings in the body, only half the job is being done. Shivering, trembling, shaking movement of different parts of the body in any directions it chooses is how one "unlearns" the pain response and "unfreezes" the brain. The mindful approach to FMS symptoms requires discipline, moment to moment awareness, and movement. If possible, gentle touch therapy which will activate the nervous system to change the negative responses of the brain should be part of this treatment.

It seems that the real cure for FMS is within ourselves. It won't be easy and I am finding that because of my age there is more for my brain to unlearn than for that of a younger person. However, there is little else out there that I can take on for treatment that I haven't tried before. I believe this is the best remedy of all.

Growing Stronger: Tending the Body

"Lack of activity destroys the good condition of
every human being, while movement and methodical
physical exercise save it and preserve it."
– Plato

Many people are searching for the ultimate regime that strengthens and improves our overall health. From the "pump iron" mantra, to Pilates videos; from parks filled with tai chi practitioners to the joggers on our sidewalks, to the yoga clubs whose numbers continue to swell, the exercise options seem endless. Those of us in chronic pain, however, are left in a state of frustration and confusion, particularly if we can sometimes barely walk!

Our health practitioners urge us to keep up with our mobility. Don't give in to the desire to lie low, we are admonished. The less you move, the less you will be able to do on a daily basis, the experts tell us. Muscles become atrophied: we understand that, but if movement brings about more pain and fatigue, how do we work through it all? More importantly, how do we decide which activity to embark upon with so many offering what each considers to be the best program?

From the website of One to One Wellness, which contains a gathering of resources for staying active even when facing chronic health challenges (www.121wellness.ca) I have borrowed information about choosing the right kind of fitness for your own body Ultimately the choice will be yours; I am not a physician and cannot recommend any of the following for you, so after consulting with a health professional, which will you choose?

Yoga

For several years, at least a decade ago, I consistently went to Iyengar yoga classes. I chose this particular style of yoga because it was a supported practice, using props such as cushions, belts, pillows and bolsters to aid those with movement challenges. I was very lucky to have had a wonderful instructor, who was very inventive with adapting poses and props for the benefit of his students. Mostly what he encouraged me to do were poses intended to relax the nervous system, with none that were harmful to my stiff muscles. I enjoyed the relaxation aspect of the practice that helped me during stressful days when I had a full-time job. Furthermore, the gentle stretches helped with mobility.

One of my favourite physiotherapists writes that yoga does not really build strength, though it increases flexibility. The downside of yoga is that increasing flexibility without increasing muscle strength can result in injury and unstable joints.

My own yoga days are over and have been for quite some time. The pain became too intense and I was not progressing towards strengthening. However, I remember fondly the relaxed state I would be in at the end of the class, lying quietly on the mat and breathing slowly. Yoga is somewhat helpful for the cardiovascular system as attention is paid to breathing, meditation, mobility and relaxation. It is quite good for hypertension, the research has shown. There is a cost factor if done in a studio and online yoga classes may also be inaccessible for those without home access to a computer.

Tai chi and qi gong

While I have not taken any tai chi, I did attend a series of qi gong classes (CFQ) qualifying me at Level One, and for awhile I practiced qi gong at home with a recording on a daily basis. I was not doing this for any of the spiritually healing aspects of the practice but for the actual movements that encouraged mobility. I am not an "energy systems" advocate as are many qi gong practitioners. For me, it was relaxing and meditative and although not intended for muscle strengthening or as a means of improving cardiovascular health, I have decided to bring forth the old recording once more as I continue on the slow burn training journey.

Both tai chi and qi gong are excellent forms of gentle movement therapy and encourage strengthening. They may even help cut down on pain medication. The mantra "motion is lotion" applies to tai chi and qi gong (along with the Feldenkrais technique). You can find practice videos easily on YouTube, if you'd like to try these movement forms at home. Moving slowly in the qi gong and tai chi postures is an excellent way to help mobility and relax the nervous system. It is particularly helpful when done in a setting with others as there is usually a general feeling that relaxation is happening in the room and attention is being paid by instructors to the persons learning the moves.

Pilates

This activity is considered by many to be the bright and shining star of modern-day physical fitness. Developed during World War 1 by Joseph Pilates for returning veterans, the intent was to use the mind to control the body. While none of us can negate the body/mind connection, it seems as though there is conflicting information regarding whether or not Pilates actually does strengthen the core muscles with the intense focus on the "core," that new buzz word. Many dispute there is a *core* of the body; it cannot be seen.

Pilates focuses on the postural muscles with exact precision and awareness of the breath. It is intended that the mind would eventually control the muscles. There is however, severe criticism of many of the untrained instructors and in particular of some of its claims.

Some of the cons of Pilates: It places too much emphasis on the abdominals and therefore can create unbalances. Furthermore, the recommended breathing exercises are harmful and can even elevate the blood pressure. Now, dear reader, please do not rebuke me for saying these things about Pilates if you are wedded to the practice. I have never done it, nor even watched it being done, nor seen a video about the system. I am merely citing information taken from the internet. There are, no doubt, many others who will swear to its value. I can only present the information which I have available. A physiotherapist I have seen believes it is a wonderful program **IF** it is practiced with a fully trained instructor on a one- to- one basis. Videos may be harmful without the attention of highly trained teachers.

Running

Those of us with fibromyalgia cannot usually run; many of us are lucky to be able to walk without pain. In my younger days I did run but as time went on, I began having so much pain that I could see that I was risking even more injury. I believe that running was very harmful to my muscular system even while I know it was helpful for my CVS and consequently my blood pressure. About this form of activity, the physiotherapist writes that it is not a flexible practice and tightness is more often the rule than the exception. He says that running can also be a nightmare for the musculoskeletal system.

While wintering in Arizona, a physical therapist told me she tells her older clients not to use even a treadmill as this too is harmful to joints and muscles. She says that long walks, especially on hard surfaces, contribute to many of the problems she sees on a daily basis. Short walks on soft surfaces are preferable and, in her words, "walking and jogging are highly overrated." My physiotherapist says of long-distance walking: "Sorry, this is not the panacea that many claim it is." Oh great! What then?

An alternative to regular walking is pool walking as it is done under ideal conditions: warm water, a quiet atmosphere, and wearing pool sneakers. There is some degree of resistance, though it is generally not considered a strengthening technique, but it *is* a plus for mobility! More expensive than walking outside in the fresh air, but definitely less harmful for the joints and muscles. The problem of accessibility and the cost of a pool membership may be prohibitive. Regular walking and running are cheap! What can a person do then if there is no pool available or the expense is too high? The challenges are numerous.

Swimming

After many years of not swimming, I decided to try it again. Phew! After two weeks I could barely move. My arms, neck, back and legs were on fire. What was I thinking? The act of swimming resulted in muscle imbalance and repetitive strain, so I ended my pool experiment

To receive the benefits of swimming, my physiotherapist says, "It's all about intensity. Swim hard or go home." Slow swimming does not appear to have much benefit for those fibromyalgia muscles. If you find swimming relaxing, though, and can make it easier on your body with floatation devices, it's worth pursuing.

Spinning

I enjoy my stationary recumbent bike, and do not experience pain when biking slowly. Though there is a risk of repetitive strain with this kind of exercise, it is balanced out by benefits to the cardiovascular system. Sure, biking slowly doesn't burn many calories or build much muscle, but it is easier on the joints than walking or jogging, and bad weather is not a factor in doing it. Stationary biking may be my ultimate form of exercise

Strength (or resistance) training

Have I found the perfect tool for my aging, painful, tired body? According to many, resistance training is *IT!* Many health and fitness experts claim that progressive resistance training is the only way to build strength slowly over time. It is excellent for the cardiovascular system, increases muscle mass, and is the only form of complete exercise. Drawbacks include the need to have a gym membership (if one chooses to practice strength training that way—gardeners, farmers, and those who do manual labour know that not all heavy lifting happens in a gym!) Furthermore, many claim that strength training is hard work and not at all fun.

If you choose to begin a resistance training regime, go slowly and make sure to leave time in between gym sessions to allow your body to recover (this applies not just to those with FMS!). As the body gets stronger, some report less pain in completing other physical activities.

Resistance training is also credited with increasing bone density, an important factor as we age and become more prone to osteoporosis.

I still don't have any definite solutions to the problem of finding the perfect exercise that won't exacerbate my condition, but I keep seeking them. Because I have lived with fibromyalgia for so many years, I sometimes think I should have been a pathfinder, yet I still don't know the right path to follow, as there are so many. As to whether or not there is one activity that fits all of us, there isn't one approach that is perfect for everyone, except perhaps gentle walks, if one is mobile.

For now, I will try to continue to pool walk a little, ride my bike, and a bit of qi gong movement, and keep hoping for a better future with less pain. I have to keep hoping that I will find the right path for me.

Eating Well with FMS

"Let food be thy medicine...."
– Hippocrates

Eating can be one of life's greatest joys. Eating for comfort can have an immediate effect on our moods, and it can often result in guilt. Eating can be a social event, or it can be done in private. Eating is sometimes only done to keep oneself alive. Eating a specific way is often done to either reduce weight or gain weight. Eating often reflects cultural and ethnic backgrounds and can be a way to show love to others. Eating and dieting go hand in hand and can bring about hope (and its opposite). So, is there hope for those who have fibromyalgia that in eating particular kinds of food, and abstaining from others, we will find relief from our symptoms? Is it realistic to give general advice to those with FMS without taking individual factors into consideration?

Along with exercise, eating specific kinds of foods has become a widely-practiced approach to good health in the 21st century. Fatty, salty and highly processed foods, as well as caffeine, colas, sugar, aspartame, preservatives and MSG should be avoided as much as possible in order to maintain a healthy lifestyle. We hear this advice often.[23]

The issue of obesity is a grave concern in our society, as is its opposite: anorexia. Furthermore, in order to enhance a healthy diet, eating locally and organically is highly recommended. But what of the people who cannot afford to buy organically, who are often so fatigued that fast foods are easier on the body than hours of food preparation, who are living on a reduced income and cannot afford fresh fruit and vegetables? The literature

---

[23] See for example *The End of Overeating,* by David A. Kessler

on fibromyalgia is replete with advice about which foods to eat and which to avoid. Rarely does the literature take into account the challenges that face the sufferer who cannot meet the requirements for healthy eating.

Eating cannot be separated from digestion; almost all people with fibromyalgia are afflicted with bowel motility issues at some point. It stands to reason that fresh fruit and raw vegetables will help with constipation, yet it is sometimes easier and cheaper to take stool softeners or laxatives than it is to buy and prepare expensive fresh foods. On the other hand, for some, diarrhea may be more of an issue than constipation, and therefore they may have to restrict high fibre foods. Indeed, for those of us with FMS, dealing with food challenges can be a full-time job.

What about those of us who are privileged enough that we can afford to eat well, but are dealing with such demons as sugar cravings? As I discuss in another section of the book, the adrenal glands are responsible for the levels of cortisol in our bodies. When we are under stress, (as many of us with FMS are, due to sleep disorders, fatigue, and pain) the high levels of cortisol in our bodies raise our blood glucose levels. It becomes a vicious cycle. With overstimulation and high levels of stress, we have a need for good nutrients to avoid adrenal exhaustion. Yet the craving for sugar and carbohydrates, not to mention other kinds of junk food, is extremely high, and the more we consume, the higher the levels of cortisol! But who can deny that these comfort foods offer at least some short-term comfort? The challenge is to find a way to deal with these high levels of cortisol in our bodies by eating foods that have been shown to be good for us. A Mediterranean diet rich in vegetables is thought to be the best approach for alleviating pain, or any diet that is filled with anti-inflammatory foods such as dark leafy greens, lean meats, and fish.

There is little doubt that eating properly to help bring down the high levels of cortisol is part of the solution to FMS pain, although not the cure. Since it is often the woman who prepares the meals, I have often asked women with FMS this question: "What works for you?" It seems to me that this is where we should begin, as there are many cultural and social variations of a healthy diet. For some who believe there are specific foods which cause discomfort, for example, wheat or dairy, then avoidance is the answer. For others, allergy testing seems to give them some answers as to which foods to avoid. Others maintain that intermittent fasting and reduction of toxins in the body help with digestion and overall well being.

The times are changing and now many men are the ones who prepare meals. I wish I had asked other genders about their meal preparations and how they addressed the issue of what to eat. Do they cook for speed, simplicity, health issues? Are they partnered or living alone? Is fibromyalgia their main concern when cooking? Are there multiple chemical sensitivities in certain foods that bother them?

Interestingly, the idea of high incidences of wheat and dairy" allergies", or perhaps more accurately, intolerances, have proliferated in Western society. The British Nutrition Foundation reports that one in five Britons now think they have a food allergy. The Foundation says that actually only a small fraction of these people actually has an allergy or intolerance to specific foods like wheat/ gluten and dairy. They base this conclusion on many worldwide studies. They regard the cultural phenomenon of food restrictions based on perceived intolerances as "trendy." Some Australian allergy specialists and others in the American Academy of Allergy, Asthma and Immunology reached similar conclusions. No doubt others would disagree with the results of these studies and reports, while continuing to believe they have wheat and dairy allergies. Those who eat only gluten-free foods or are vegetarian or vegan are no longer a minority.

Even if there isn't as high an incidence of food allergies or sensitivities as it would seem, if people feel better by giving them up, then perhaps it is due to the placebo effect. As has often been shown, the placebo effect can be very helpful and should never be discounted.

I personally do not seem to have wheat or dairy intolerances, and I often enjoy a chai latte. I eat whole grains, particularly early in the day and wheat does not cause any discomfort for me. However, I know many people with FMS and chemical sensitivities who restrict their diets dramatically. We all have to do whatever we think is helpful to us in our daily struggles. One eating program does not fit all. Probably the best advice is to eat in moderation, with a well-balanced diet and to avoid fad diets that promise cures.

Finally, some advice from someone who has engaged in emotional eating. It is well known that with stress one's body increases its production of insulin. This can lead to a vicious cycle of eating "comfort" foods, mainly consisting of carbohydrates and sugar, which inflame the muscles and cause those of us with FMS to have more pain. We then eat more comfort food because it brings temporary comfort, perpetuating a vicious circle. We have to be alert to the foods that cause our symptoms to become worse, in particular refined sugar: candy, caffeine, cookies, cakes, and ice cream. These sugars are probably **the** worst for muscle pain, so we must avoid them at all costs. It is an ongoing challenge that I personally struggle with on a daily basis!

Talking About Our Pain

"We also often add to our own pain and suffering by
being overly sensitive, over-reacting to minor things,
and sometimes taking things too personally."
– Tenzin Gyatso, The 14th Dalai Lama

One of the challenges that people with fibromyalgia grapple with is trying to describe their pain to others. Descriptors such as "aching", "raw," "ragged," "searing," "blistering," "shocking," or "nagging" do not always convey the message to health professionals and loved ones; the list of adjectives is endless. The vocabulary for pain is not precise and it can be a daunting task to find the right words. Even more frustrating is that the nature of the pain itself changes, sometimes from hour to hour or day to day. Equally problematic to describe are the areas of the body where pain attacks, as they can move from place to place or occur in several areas of the body simultaneously.

Pain research has been built upon the premise that there are scales which can measure the degree of suffering. We commonly use this language in our everyday talk in a variety of ways; for example, we ask of others, "On a scale of 0 to 10, how did you rate the movie?" When it comes to intangibles like our emotions, surveys abound with rating scales presumed to quantify subjective characteristics such as happiness, depression, grief, and other emotions, along with our attitudes, beliefs and values. We have a strong desire to categorize the subjective elements of our nature and personality in an objective fashion. It is assumed that we could simplify our lives if we all experienced life in the same way, without taking into account our personal circumstances, age, gender, race, class, and personality, among many other variables. If we could categorize people according to scales, (usually called

Likert scales) it would help us in quantifying such subjective characteristics as fibromyalgia pain. However, is this truly possible?

In an issue of the *Journal of General Internal Medicine* the results of one research article showed that rating systems failed nearly one third of the time. While the study acknowledges that pain is subjective, its authors also suggest that there is reluctance on the part of some people to admit to their pain while others may exaggerate it. Pain also comes and goes and it is therefore difficult to rate.

Having spoken with hundreds of fibromyalgia sufferers, it has not been my observation that people are hesitant to admit to their pain. In fact, knowing that I too have fibromyalgia, they are always ready to discuss the ever-present pain but they often keep silent around those who do not have the same experience. Those of us with FMS simply do not want to sound as though we are whiners or constant complainers to "outsiders," and equally as important, the pain issues are so complex that language becomes difficult. Pain is invisible and talking about it, particularly to those who believe it is all in one's head, is very silencing.

As I discuss in my earlier book, there are many components to the experience of pain; age, culture, race and gender all play a significant role in how much we are able to share with researchers or health professionals regarding pain. Men must be stoic and generally not complain or else they are afraid of being thought of as a "sissy," while women have traditionally suffered in silence. With the current higher rate of transgendered persons, it would be interesting to know if there is more or less likelihood of discussing pain with their physicians.

One of the Black women I interviewed in my previous book said that it is not acceptable for a Black woman to complain about pain; she must be seen to be a "strong Black woman." Another woman I interviewed came from Germany where she said to speak of suffering was to show weakness. Most of the women acknowledged that when men reported pain, the doctors took notice, but if they complained they were not as well attended to and often felt ashamed of even mentioning their suffering.

When I was in my menopause years, everything I reported to my doctor regarding fibromyalgia was attributed to menopause.

In the late 1980s, the Fibromyalgia Impact Questionnaire was developed to help quantify the symptoms of this syndrome. This rating scale is freely available for all who want to use it and was reported in 1991 by researchers Burckhardt, Clark and Bennett in the *Journal of Rheumatology*. Interestingly, pain is a somewhat small component of the questionnaire as are other factors such as fatigue. Other scales like the Visual Analogue Scale whereby a patient marks on a line the amount of pain one experiences ranging from "no pain" to "very severe pain" are also commonly used to measure the symptom. But to what extent are these rating scales accurate? It is admirable that researchers are attempting to find ways to measure pain. But is this possible using numbers that depict quantity rather than finding ways to explore quality? As previously mentioned, it is as though one person's specific circumstances were all the same as anyone else's with this condition. We know that pain in fibromyalgia can change from hour to hour or day to day. It is not a static linear process. Pain is like ice cream; it comes in different flavours.

We cannot yet adequately describe overwhelming pain and fatigue and the myriad of other often agonizing symptoms that accompany the syndrome. But there are moments of relief and there is hope that life can be lived more fully. Mindfulness, vibroacoustic music (especially harp), and music therapy hold out much promise for the treatment of chronic FMS pain—please see the book by Daniel J. Levitin *This is Your Brain on Music* which has led me to believe that music therapy might be helpful for people with fibromyalgia.

Conclusion

I wonder now what is left to say that I haven't written about over my many years of living with fibromyalgia. I hope that I have unravelled the complexity of this syndrome and provided food for thought to those of us living in constant pain and enduring a host of other challenges. I can't pretend to know all the answers and yet I feel very sure that the suggestions I have made about living a better quality of life can and should be incorporated into our daily lives.

There isn't anyone out there with specific answers, medications, or strategies which will help us unless we are willing to help ourselves. The struggles are many, but we are valiant people with great gifts to offer with our intuitions, insights and empathy. It is the readers who have commented on my blogs, the researchers of the brain, and other health professionals who have awakened in me an awareness about becoming the experts of our own lives. I owe you so much.

May you feel a sense of empowerment and peace as you walk the path of self- healing from fibromyalgia.

To my wonderful editor Elizabeth Pierce I owe great appreciation. Thank you for all you did to help me complete this project. You are an editor par excellence.

La vie est belle

Appendix: Resources

The following is a list of books, websites, and videos on topics related to fibromyalgia that I have found helpful.

Neuroplasticity

Daniel Amen, *Change Your Brain*

Norman Doidge, *The Brain That Changes Itself* and *The Brain's Way of Healing*

Barbara Arrowsmith-Young, *The Woman who Changed her Brain*

Mindfulness

Jon Kabat-Zinn, *Full Catastrophe Living*

Craig Hassed, *Know Thyself*

Pema Chödrön, *When Things Fall Apart*

Mark Williams/Danny Penman, *Mindfulness: An Eight-Week Plan for Finding Peace in a Frantic World*

Chronic pain

David Butler and Lorimer Moseley, *Explain Pain*

Toni Bernhard, *How to Live Well with Chronic Pain and Illness* and *How to be Sick*

Elaine Scarry, *The Body in Pain*

Bronnie Lennox Thompson blog, https://healthskills.wordpress.com

Chronic fatigue syndrome

Dr. Eleanor Stein, http://www.eleanorsteinmd.ca

Healing from trauma

Peter Levine, *Waking the Tiger*

Bessel van der Kolk, *The Body Keeps the Score*

Anxiety and depression

Daniel Smith, *Monkey Mind*

Scott Stossel, *My Age of Anxiety*

Eleanor Morgan, *Anxiety for Beginners*

Wendy Suzuki, *Good Anxiety*

Williams, Kabat-Zinn, et al, *The Mindful Way through Depression*

Tara Brach, *Radical Acceptance*

Emotional/nervous system regulation

Dr. Richie Davidson, "The Emotional Life of Your Brain," YouTube video https://www.youtube.com/watch?v=GnwhoVR4fCw

Diane Jacobs "Know Your Nervous System," YouTube video https://www.youtube.com/watch?v=LCsvOqag9eI&t=20s

Diane Jacobs website: https://www.dermoneuromodulation.com/

Dr. Suzanne LaCombe, "Self-Regulation Therapy," http://www.myshrink.com.

Mind and body

Robert Baer, *The Body Bears the Burden*

Sandra and Matthew Blakeslee, *The Body Has a Mind of Its Own*

Deric Bownds, *The Biology of Mind: Origins and Structures of Mind, Brain and Consciousness*

John Sarno, *The Divided Mind: The Epidemic of Mind-Body Disorders*

Memory

Maria Konnikova, *Mastermind*

Lars Clausen, *Fibromyalgia Relief* ("memory reconsolidation")

Harvard Health, Harvard Medical School website, "Memory" https://www.health.harvard.edu/topics/memory

Cannabis

Dr. Julie Holland, *The Pot Book: A Complete Guide to Cannabis*

M. Backes, *Cannabis Pharmacy*

J. Groopman, "Marijuana: The High and the Low," in *A New Leaf: The End of Cannabis Prohibition*

Sensitivity

Elaine Aron, *The Highly Sensitive Person*

Ted Zeff, *The Highly Sensitive Person's Guide*

Acceptance and commitment therapy (ACT)

Steven Hayes and Spencer Smith, *Get Out of Your Mind and Into Your Life*

Dr. Steven Hayes' website contains a number of useful worksheets and other resources: https://stevenchayes.com/my-act-toolkit/

Music therapy

Daniel J. Levitin, *This is Your Brain on Music*

Storytelling

Will Storr, *The Science of Storytelling*

Nicholas Epley, *Mindwise*

Itching

Dr. Zhou-Feng Chen, https://itch.wustl.edu/

Dizziness/vertigo

Mayo Clinic, "Dizziness," https://www.mayoclinic.org/diseases-conditions/dizziness/diagnosis-treatment/drc-20371792

Carol Foster MS vertigo treatment, YouTube video, https://www.youtube.com/watch?v=mQR6b7CAiqk

Printed in the United States
by Baker & Taylor Publisher Services